With the Wind
and the Waves

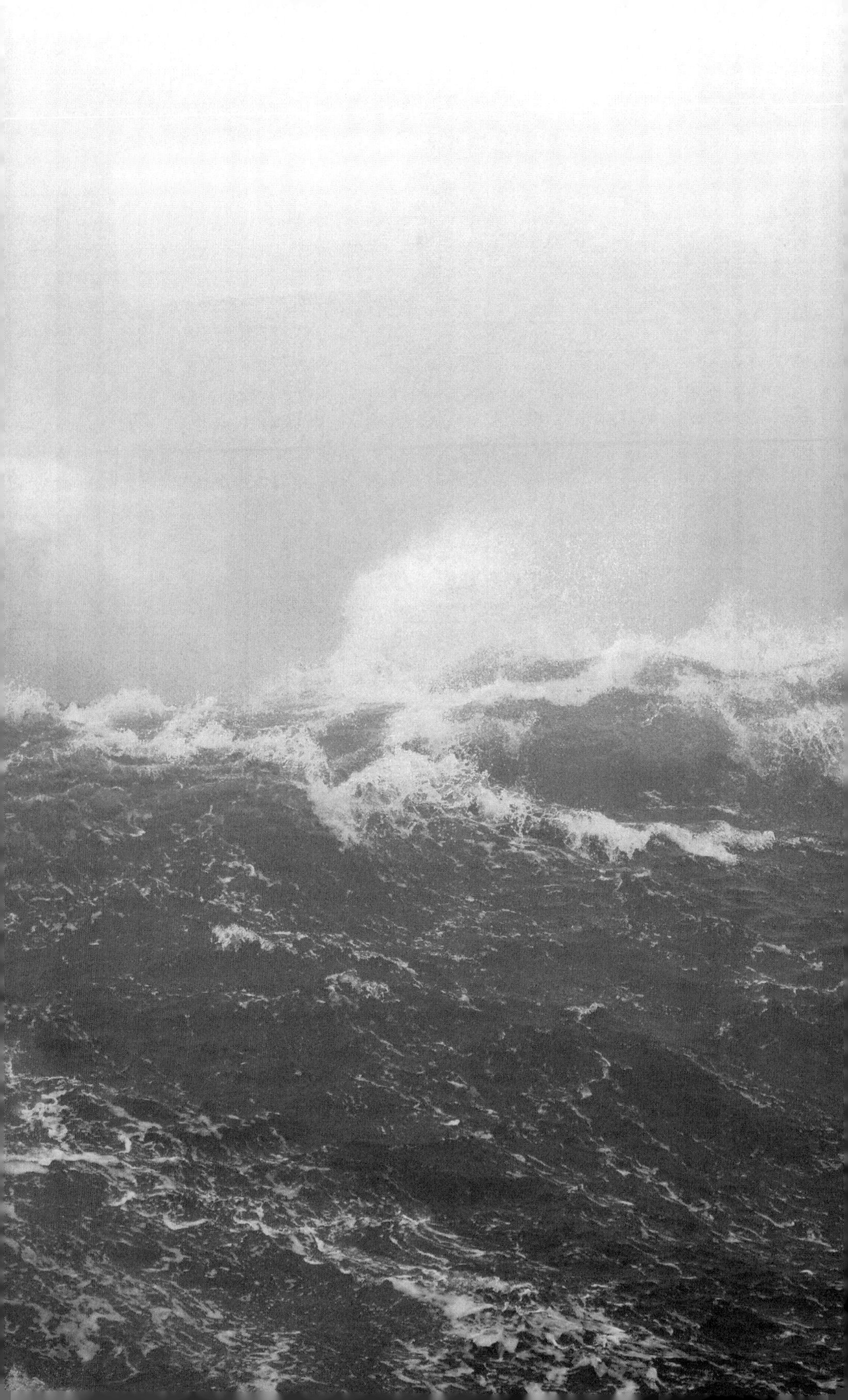

With the Wind and the Waves

A Guide to Mental Health Practices in Alaska Native Communities

Ray M. Droby

University of Alaska Press
Fairbanks, Alaska

The views expressed in this manual are those of the author and not necessarily those of the Norton Sound Health Corporation (NSHC) or Indian Health Service (IHS) of the United States Public Health Service (USPHS).

The author has received no monies from this publication. All author rights and royalties have been transferred to the tribal agency of the Norton Sound Health Corporation.

Text © 2020 University of Alaska Press
Published by
University of Alaska Press
P.O. Box 756240
Fairbanks, AK 99775-6240

Cover and interior design by Paula Elmes.

With the Wind and the Waves was originally published in 2000 by Norton Sound Health Corporation. It is now redesigned by the University of Alaska Press and reprinted with substantial updates and additions.

Library of Congress Cataloging-in-Publication Data

Names: Droby, Ray M., author.
Title: With the wind and the waves : a guide for mental health practices in Alaska Native communities / by Ray M. Droby.
Description: Fairbanks : University of Alaska Press, [2020] | Includes bibliographical references and index.
Identifiers: LCCN 2020004015 (print) | LCCN 2020004016 (ebook) | ISBN 9781602234161 (paperback) | ISBN 9781602234178 (ebook)
Subjects: LCSH: Alaska Natives—Mental health services. | Psychiatry, Transcultural—Alaska.
Classification: LCC RC451.5.I5 D76 2020 (print) | LCC RC451.5.I5 (ebook) | DDC 616.89009798—dc23
LC record available at https://lccn.loc.gov/2020004015
LC ebook record available at https://lccn.loc.gov/2020004016

To the survivors of sexual abuse across the State of Alaska:

women, children, and men.

May your voices be heard forevermore.

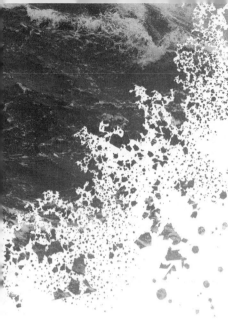

Contents

We will be heard, in the wind, on the water,

and in the quiet dignity of our old ones:

The people speak: Will YOU listen?

—*Robin A. LaDue (1994)*

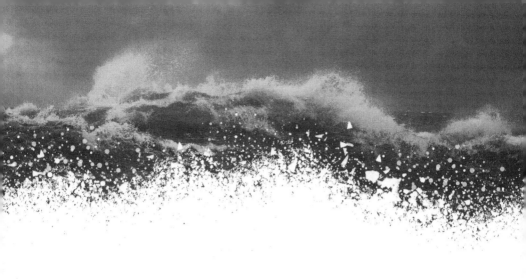

Preface

This is a revision of my previous book, *With the Wind and the Waves*, published by the Norton Sound Health Corporation in 2000. Some material from the earlier publication is included verbatim in this revised version—most notably my ocean journey and what I learned from it and the "lesson" I learned in my Head Start visit.

As one Native mental health professional once explained to me: "There are no recipes for interacting within a Native community." Alaska's Behavioral Health Aide (BHA) Program, designed to promote behavioral health and wellness in Alaska Native individuals, families, and communities, employs village-based counselors who are predominantly Native and live in their Native community. There are thirteen regional Native health corporations in Alaska. They provide a variety of medical and mental health services to their centralized localities or hub communities and the surrounding Native communities in their catchment vicinity.

In the Bering Strait region, Nome serves as the hub to fifteen out-lying Native communities encompassing a vast 23,000-square-mile area including the Bering Sea, Norton Sound, St. Lawrence Island, and the Seward Peninsula. Outlying Native communities range in population from approximately 750 residents (the largest) to 110 residents (the smallest). These communities are predominantly accessible only by small plane. Village-based counselors work alongside licensed mental health professionals, who are often non-Native and itinerate from Nome to serve the outlying Native villages. Although behavioral health aides receive culturally relevant training and education, no such training is conducted with non-Native mental health professionals who work in Native villages. Further, empirical research is lacking regarding guidelines for non-Native mental health professionals living and/or working within Alaska Native communities. Historically, it has been left to the non-Native therapist—often new to Alaska from the Lower 48—to figure out a culturally sensitive approach to mental health work within Native communities. This book aims to provide a model for non-Native mental health professionals working and/or living in Alaska Native communities. I hope that Native mental health providers will also find its material useful.

In this book, I use the terms "Bering Strait region" and "Norton Sound" interchangeably and sometimes in isolation. References to Norton Sound, for example, recognize Native communities specific to that locale—but, again, Norton Sound is part of the Bering Strait region.

This guide begins with principles gleaned from my experiential journey on the ocean. I present theoretical and practical insights, coupled with a flexible template for performing mental health work with Alaska Natives, stemming from over two decades of living and working in four Native communities in the Bering Strait region and living and working in the hub community of Nome. With over 200 Native villages in Alaska, comprising about 16 percent of Alaska's population, the Native communities of Alaska are both similar and diverse. The flexibility of the factors described here for performing mental health work in Alaska Native villages aims to capture the complexity of working with Alaska Natives amid such similarity and diversity. In the same spirit, the factors delineated hold promising applicability to Lower 48 Native Americans, particularly in light of the trauma of colonization.

Finally, although this book was initially written with non-Native mental health providers in mind, it does not exclude Native mental health providers. As Dr. Tina Woods explains (see page 10), there are reasons to include Native mental health providers. So, my references to "mental health professionals" include non-Native and Native mental health providers. I do, however, refer to "non-Native mental health professionals" when emphasis toward this group of individuals is indicated.

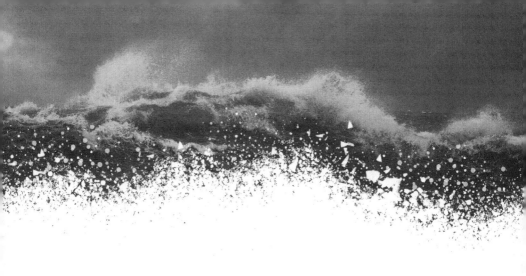

Acknowledgments

Heartfelt appreciation extends to the Norton Sound Health Corporation, serving the Native communities of the Bering Strait region and Norton Sound, for approving this publication. I also extend my appreciation to the Indian Health Service of the United States Public Health Service for providing me with the opportunity to serve in rural Alaska. I thank my village-based colleague, Ward Walker, for his inspiring and selfless devotion to the Native peoples of the Bering Strait region and Norton Sound. I acknowledge my former village-based colleagues, Gladys Pete and Alice Fitka, who together we shared many wonderful projects in their respective communities and whose tireless work will always be remembered and admired. I thank my current village-based colleague, behavioral health practitioner Elvina Turner, whose grounded presence, wisdom, support, and knowledge of her community was and is greatly appreciated. I will always remember the late Teresa Perry who exemplified the behavioral health practitioner role. Teresa was a tremendous advocate for her people: she worked with everyone in her community including its leaders, school personnel, and all ages of people with a variety of presenting problems. She worked to decrease the stigma of mental health by performing regular presentations on emotional well-being in school classrooms encompassing all grades. She did evening support groups with young teenagers. She engaged the youth in her community with planning and implementing summer camps related to cultural activities such as subsistence. One of her many talents that I admired her for was her persistent effort toward insuring that the Elders always received optimum integrated healthcare. Teresa passed on too young and is missed by many. I thank my editor, Nate Bauer, and his staff at the University of Alaska Press, for their commitment to this manuscript. I thank the Alaska Native Tribal Health Consortium for their work on many levels toward promoting the strengths of Alaska Natives and their communities; I give particular appreciation for the support I received from Carolyn Craig and Xiomara Owens. I extend deepest gratitude to my friend Mel Riley, whose knowledge of Native American history and his respect for Native cul-tures was educational and inspiring. Thanks to the behavioral health aides and behavioral health practitioners of the Bering Strait region and Norton Sound for their commitment to their communities and self-determination. I am grateful to Donna Barr of Shishmaref, who kept me updated on the progress of her community's efforts toward relocation. To Dr. Pamela Hays I express my deepest appreciation for her helpful, pertinent feedback regarding the organization of this manuscript and its contents. For their support of this publication and their wonderful insight and feedback, I greatly extend thanks to Drs. Iva GreyWolf, Jordan Lewis, and Tina Woods. To Jay David: your clinical validation, insight and encouragement were much appreciated. I owe an enormous amount of thanks to Sigrid Brudie and her staff at the Alaska Medical Library, University of Alaska, Anchorage: your prompt attention to the references I needed kept me in a productive state of flow; I could not have completed this manuscript without your reliable, competent assistance. I thank my wife, Hang, and my sons, Bryan and Conrad, who tolerated my time away from them on weekends and evenings to write my book. To the Native communities of the Bering Strait region and Norton Sound: you have educated me in so many different ways and have enriched my life immeasurably. Thank you to the Elders, who fervently share their culture with the youth of their communities and make their voices heard for generations to come. Finally, to all the traditional healers who carry on the ancient practices to maintain peace and balance among their people.

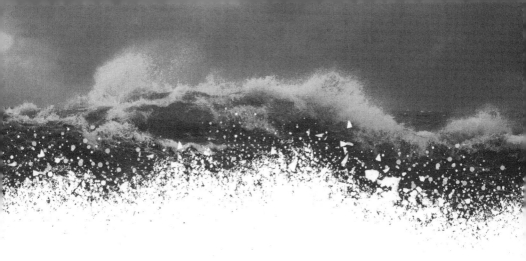

CHAPTER ONE

With the Wind and the Waves: A Guide for Mental Health Practices in Alaska Native Communities

Six weeks after moving to the Central Yup'ik village of Stebbins in 1997, where I was asked to work with their village-based counseling program, I ventured out in my canoe one October evening after work and headed for Stuart Island about two miles off the coast. I had been told by one villager to forget about going to the island in October due to the intense storms that came at this time of year. An Elder, too, told me that the water was "heavy water" at this time of the year, and therefore not good for traveling. Moreover, everyone warned me that when there was a strong wind I should not enter the water. But the Bering Sea was calm this evening and I made camp uneventfully on the island just as the sun was beginning to set. A campfire, a steak dinner, and a full moon made the experience magical.

It rained intermittently during the night. But the next morning the sun shone brightly—ushering in a cold autumn day coupled with a brisk wind from the north. I spent most of the day exploring the tiny portion of the island I had landed upon before packing up for the return voyage to Stebbins. Since I was on the south side of Stuart Island, I was protected from the high winds and easily negotiated the southern coast of the island. I stopped, however, on the last peninsula to scout the final two miles to Stebbins across Stephens Pass, a deep channel of ocean water lying between the island and the mainland.[1]

The channel looked passable in spite of the high winds from the north. The waves did not appear to be swelling too high, and I observed no whitecaps. I knew, too, that my canoe was quite capable of forging Class III rapids, and these waves did not even approach that intensity. Yet the high winds worried me. They were a menacing combination with the frigid ocean. So, I compromised: I reasoned that I would paddle out about a quarter mile, and if the waves and wind became overwhelming, I would return to the island and camp there for another night.

I headed out with my plan settled in my mind—making a diagonal cut toward the coastline since the wind would not allow me direct passage to Stebbins. About a quarter mile out, the sea and the wind suddenly appeared to turn on me. Seemingly from nowhere, I was assaulted with three-foot swells and a constant blast of wind that funneled through Stephens Pass, between the island and the mainland. I immediately turned the boat around and paddled as hard as I could back toward the island. But I was held fast in a peculiar current and winds that were pushing my canoe, situated parallel against the waves, out toward deeper water, the open ocean, and farther from land.

I turned the boat back toward the coastline and tried paddling, but I was held firmly in place. I turned it again back toward the island, but I was also held firmly in this position. I simply could not move backward or forward. And when I tried paddling, the canoe

---

1 Geographically, Stebbins is on an island—separated by the St. Michael Canal from the true mainland, surrounding it to the south and east; however, this text will refer to Stebbins and its coastline as constituting the "mainland."

became ominously unstable. The only progress I was making was being pushed parallel from the island out into the open ocean, farther and farther from land.

Exhausted, I held up my paddle, waving it in the wind, hoping that someone in Stebbins would see my predicament and come rescue me in a motorboat. But I knew I was two miles away and appeared only as a dot from the shoreline. I tried holding the metal portion of my paddle in the sunlight, hoping the aluminum shaft would glisten—offering a beacon to those possibly watching from land. Stephen Crane's "The Open Boat" flashed in my mind, reminding me that life can be so ironic and indifferent: encapsulated in happiness one moment, then precariously close to death the next.

I am going to die, I thought to myself. A feeling of resignation began to settle within me. Even though I was wearing warm clothing and a personal flotation vest, and my canoe was equipped with its own flotation gear, I expected the waves to soon begin swamping the boat. I would get wet and die of hypothermia, lying on the hull of my overturned canoe like the people of the *Titanic* clinging to debris in the Atlantic Ocean. I could not feel my legs because I had been kneeling in the canoe for a long time. I had the macabre thought that at least my legs would not feel hypothermic pain; I only had to deal with my upper body dying from an icy bath.

I quit paddling. Fighting the current and the wind was useless. I had no option but to simply stop what I was doing. The harder I tried to escape, the more danger I placed myself in. It was as if the wind and the waves demanded that I dance with them. And though I was not in the mood to participate in the dance, I could not avoid it. So I simply remained kneeling in my canoe, letting the waves and the wind carry me as they wished. I had given up hope for any help from the mainland. I was on my own.

The waves increased to four-foot swells and were beginning to crest. It was unnerving to watch each frothing wave approach my boat from the side, so I avoided looking at them altogether. I reasoned that if a wave was going to swamp my canoe, I could not do anything about it. Therefore, it was pointless to terrify myself by scrutinizing each oncoming surge of water. Instead, I focused on two canoe tips I had been taught: keep your paddle in the water at all times to increase the canoe's stability, and stay low in the boat to maintain a low center of gravity. If I were going to be swamped, the waves would have to do all the work for me.

Time passed. I have no idea how long I was stuck in this position, but the sun facing me from the west was clearly descending on the horizon. I was prepared to stay in this impassive posture through the night.

I do not know to whom I prayed out there. It may have been to my delusions or some spiritual presence lingering there in the waves and the wind. But I know I prayed. And I promised whoever was with me at that moment that if I survived I would write about how this ocean experience paralleled my work in the Native village of Stebbins.

During the time I was held captive, moving with the waves and the wind, my thoughts became acutely focused on my work in Stebbins. I regretted that my work would be cut short. More poignantly, I realized how my predicament paralleled my work in the village. I reflected on the history of Alaska Natives, how Anglo/European influence rendered an entire culture and nation of people traumatized in multiple ways. And then I thought about how an outside mental health professional such as myself can make things worse when not considering such a history. We can come into communities with good intentions and be zealots in our efforts to effect positive change. Yet often we are met with resistance. And if we fail to realize that such resistance is frequently grounded in unresolved trauma in the people we are trying to help, we can become frustrated and, worse, judgmental. As outsiders, we can become mired in a state of stagnation and emotional burnout—disappointed that our apparent good efforts are not being appreciated by the people we came to help.

In such a state of emotional helplessness, we may try harder and harder to push our good projects. To ward off the thought that maybe we are really doing the wrong thing, we can begin to think that we are superior in some way and that the Native people might need to be pushed a little bit more. We can become so zealous with savior attitudes, that we lose touch with basic common sense and practicing kindness toward our fellow humankind. Instead of focusing on the things we can do, we judge Native people as "apathetic" or "in denial." In the end, the relationship between the outside helper and Native people suffers horribly, and nothing is accomplished. In fact, our presence may make things worse.

The dance of the ocean and the wind returned to me. I was amazed that I was still afloat. I did not understand why the growing waves did not fill my boat with water and sink it. This still remains a mystery to me. Yet each time a wave approached the side of my canoe—the top of it cresting with white froth—my boat was suddenly lifted up, and the surge of water passed harmlessly underneath.

I knew I could never reach the island by paddling against the wind, even though it was less than half a mile away. And I knew I could never reach Stebbins. Clearly, my goal of paddling to either point of land was fruitless. But, before darkness fell, I was determined to try once more to turn my canoe around and head for the coastline—head for any piece of land I could possibly land upon, even if it meant paddling to the mouth of the Yukon River sixty miles south.

Between the assault of the swells, I managed to turn the boat around.

This time, however, I pointed my canoe more in the direction and rhythm of the wind and the waves and paddled. To my surprise, I began moving. Initially, I thought I was delusional—only imagining that I was moving when I was simply sitting still. But I gauged my progress with the mainland on my left and clearly saw that I was, indeed, moving forward. I had been cut loose from the death grip that had rooted me in one place. I knew that the path I was taking was not going to land me in Stebbins, but I would make it somewhere down the coastline south of the village. I would make it if the waves did not swamp me.

By now, the waves had grown to six-foot swells. As much as I tried to ignore them, I could not. They simply were too big and too imposing. There were moments when my canoe would catch a swell in just the right position—sending me at incredible speed through a chute of water like a surfer catching a wave in Hawaii. At other times, I had to stop paddling and wait for a whitecap to pass underneath me or assault me from the side while I held my paddle firmly in the water. Sometimes a wave would fall over the side of the canoe. Overall, though, I did not take on significant water.

When the waves did not coax me forward, it was slow progress. In spite of moving with the wind and the flow of the waves, paddling was still an arduous task. During these times, the words of the Elder returned to me: "heavy water." Seeing sand lying in a puddle of water in the bottom of my boat made me realize how the autumn storms had churned up high concentrations of silt. "Heavy water" was, in fact, a very accurate description.

Twilight descended. I continued to engage in a rhythmic pattern of racing down six-foot waves and stopping to allow a whitecap to pass beneath me or brace my canoe as a frothing crest of water assaulted the left side of my boat. I was getting seasick. But I continued paddling and stopping as I negotiated the only pathway the waves and the wind allowed me to pursue. If the waves did not get any bigger, I was beginning to think for the first time that I actually had a chance to reach the coastline. I was beginning to think that I might be able to survive.

There came a time when I looked to the left and realized there were no more waves coming at me. I looked around at the water. Although it was being ruffled by the high winds, it possessed no huge swells. I gazed ahead and saw the muddy coastline about a half mile away. I stuck my paddle down into the water and discovered that it was only two feet deep. I am going to make it, I thought. Tears flooded my eyes. I did not know it at the time, but I had landed six miles south of Stebbins. But in that moment, it did not matter. All I knew was that I was going to reach land. I was going to live.

Resistance, I came to appreciate in my dance with the wind and the waves, is natural. There are many Alaska Natives harboring hurt and pain from their oppressed histories. Many people, even entire families and communities, exist on a plateau of apparent stagnation where immediate positive change is not forthcoming. This is not a Native phenomenon. It is a human phenomenon. Moreover, maybe "resistance" really is not resistance at all but rather more of a reflection of faulty ways of working with the people we are trying to help. And maybe resistance, too, is an attempt by people to communicate the need to move in a different direction.

I once worked at a state prison in California where I had a White Vietnam war veteran as a client. He came to his weekly sessions religiously—in spite of having no need to pacify his parole board because he was slated to leave the prison in less than one year. He was a complex man with post-traumatic stress disorder who hid behind large, dark-tinted eyeglasses. Yet in the year I worked with him, he slowly revealed the pain he harbored within: the pain of being a prisoner of war and watching the men under his command being tortured to death by the Viet Cong. He preferred to sleep during the day since the night terrified him—reminding him of the gruesome treatment he had suffered while being held prisoner. The psychiatrist who supplied him with anti-anxiety medication was thoroughly frustrated with his apparent lack of progress. One day she angrily told me: "That man needs to grow up. The war's been over for twenty years!"

For many people, however, the war is not over. Residual emotions and memories from past traumas—some dramatic, some more subtle—remain lodged in an individual's sense of self. With proper help, traumatized people can gain meaning and mastery over unresolved pain to the extent that such pain can diminish and not be so intrusive and pronounced in their lives. For people helping to heal those in pain, we need to be patient and understand that humans cope and manage their lives the best they can.

Where, then, does this leave the outsider trying to facilitate change in Native communities? As my experience on the ocean taught me, I need to respect and move at the pace of the village and its people. If I do not respect this flow, I can create more problems, and my presence becomes another example of European encroachment. The last thing Native people need is outsiders telling them how to be human. Our work is better served by respecting the rhythm of a Native community and moving in directions it will allow us to go. A community, like an ocean, has avenues which we can negotiate together to effect positive change.

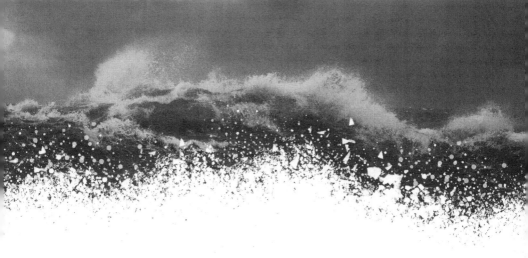

CHAPTER TWO

Guiding Principles for Mental Health Professionals Working in Alaska Native Communities

Four guiding principles fuel the infrastructure for mental health professionals working in Alaska Native communities. Embodied within this framework is a particular emphasis on non-Native practitioners working alongside village-based personnel, coupled with the need to understand and accept Native people for who they are, working with them on an individual and community level. Following my experience on the ocean, this framework emphasizes that mental health professionals must flow along with what is given in a Native community. Further, although my reference to "mental health professionals" is often intended for non-Native mental health providers, this does not exclude Native mental health providers for the following reasons: (1) some American Indian providers who move to Alaska to practice in rural/remote Alaska villages are not familiar with Alaska Native culture or the history of trauma experienced by Alaska Native people; and (2) some Alaska Native providers may not be familiar with their culture or history (e.g., they were raised outside of Alaska and not connected to the culture); this is not uncommon since most of the Alaska Native history is not taught in school but rather learned through Elders and the practice of oral tradition.[2]

Because mental health professionals come from diverse clinical backgrounds and orientations, we need to operate on some common ground. We can have many tools and techniques, but if we do not have sound principles underlying them, then our behavior may be skewed in an unhealthy or meaningless direction. If we have central principles permeating our work, then our presence in rural Alaska communities is more likely to be positive and not harmful as it has been historically for many non-Native outsiders entering Alaska Native communities.

The following principles are intended as guidance for rural mental health workers in Native communities.

1. Self-Determination Is an Inalienable Right for Alaska Natives

Self-determination is not an exclusive Native need or phenomenon. It is a fundamental human need and basic right. Humans have the right to assert themselves and make their own choices and decisions. Moreover, we must believe in the human capacity to heal, to learn, to function effectively. If we do not endorse the principle of self-determination in our work, then I seriously question our motives for working with Alaska Natives and for doing mental health work in general. Are we out here for an "experience"? For a Peace Corps–type of adventure? To write an article for *National Geographic*? To resolve some inner midlife crisis? To get our student loans paid off?

---

2   I thank Dr. Tina Woods, Chief Administrative Officer, Tanadgusix Corporation, village corporation of St.Paul Island, for her input on these important points.

To get in touch with our inner child while we work amid the great Alaska wilderness?

Consistent with the perspective of self-determination, LaDue (1994) asserts that Native people "do not need any more people who want to 'do something for us,' 'rescue' our poor children, 'save our souls'" (106). She contends that non-Native mental health professionals must pursue work within Native communities "with compassion, understanding, humility, and a desire to learn" (101). So how do we define ourselves, our roles, within the context of self-determination and Alaska Native communities? As Bopp (1994) entertains, are we an educator? A facilitator? An adviser? A mirror? A coach? A friend?

LaDue elucidates the bizarre situation non-Native mental health providers enter into when they work within Native communities. Indeed, there are many potential forms of colonization—some subtle and some more dramatic—that attempt to impose agendas upon Indigenous people: non-Native mental health providers using "evidence-based" treatment programs; schools employing Lower 48 curriculum in Native classrooms; missionaries indoctrinating Natives in Christian theology; scholars conducting research; and various agencies from outside cities attempting to promote economic development and other goals within Native communities.

Mental health providers need to be cognizant of imposing programs that are not culturally consistent. If we impose agendas—similar to how I wanted to impose my agenda of paddling to Stebbins without considering the wind and the waves—our efforts can be unproductive and harmful. Anything we do that does not embody the principle of human self-determination is likely to be counterproductive to Alaska Natives. In this manner, we come to emulate the historical behavior of colonizers at the expense of Native empowerment. And, in this fashion, we are likely to join the legacy of our non Native ancestors who came to the land of Alaska without respecting the sovereignty of Alaska Natives. We are likely to contribute to the historical oppression of Alaska Natives in subtle and sometimes more severe ways.

2. Native Self-Determination Is Best Promoted Through Decentralized Mental Health Services

Decentralized mental health services carry the spirit of an "upriver" approach to dealing with mental health problems. Instead of waiting for crises to occur and to receive them "downriver," resources are placed where such crises occur in the hope of providing support to prevent them from taking place.

In the 1990s, Nome's Norton Sound Health Corporation implemented a village-based counseling program that provided one Native counselor to each of the surrounding fifteen Native communities. This program continues today. Previously, a Nome-based non-Native mental health professional would fly out to a Native community on an itinerant basis, approximately once a month for a two- or three-day visit. The village-based counseling program, referred to as the Behavioral Health Aide (BHA) Program, is governed by the Community Health Aide Program Certification Board, unique to Alaska and the Alaska Tribal Health System (ATHS). It is modeled after the successful Community Health Aide Program, which has provided village-based primary care services throughout Alaska since the 1960s.

The BHA Program, federally recognized in 2008, provides a breadth of behavioral health services to Native villages across a continuum of care (i.e., prevention, early intervention, crisis response, and postvention). Behavioral health aides (BHAs), often Native individuals who live in remote Native communities, have different levels of certification. BHAs provide a broad range of practice based on their certification level, including community prevention, education, and wellness activities; behavioral health screening; screening and brief intervention; short-term crisis stabilization; individual, group, and family therapy; substance abuse assessment and treatment; case management and referrals; and peer support services. At the highest level of certification, behavioral health practitioners (BHPs) can provide expanded and more complex services such as in-depth counseling and supervision of BHAs at a lower level of certification.

BHA training and educational requirements are met primarily, but not exclusively, through three programs: the University of Alaska Fairbanks Rural Human Services (RHS), the Alaska Native Tribal Health Consortium (ANTHC), and the Regional Alcohol and Drug Abuse Counseling Training (RADACT). The BHA Program is facilitated through ANTHC's Behavioral Health Department in collaboration with the Behavioral Health Academic Review Committee (BHARC), a subcommittee of the Tribal Behavioral Health Directors.[3]

The BHA Program supports Native self-determination in mental health and substance abuse services through promoting behavioral health and wellness in Alaska Native people by training and educating behavioral health aides. Further, it is grounded in culturally sensitive values that embrace the emotional, physical, spiritual, social, and cultural well-being of individuals, their families, and the communities where they live. Native individuals and Native communities serving their own people and their mental health and substance abuse issues is the vision of the future.

3. The Role of the Mental Health Professional Imparts a Co-Participatory and Background Presence

The role of the mental health professional, particularly those who are non-Native, must be consistent with Native self-determination. The licensed clinician working with BHAs/BHPs must behave in a manner that reflects the values of Native self-determination. It is not

---

3   I thank Carolyn Craig, ANTHC training director for the CHA Program, and Xiomara Owens, ANTHC training director for the BHA Program, for their contributions to this section.

enough to simply articulate such a philosophy without demonstrating it through our demeanor.

If we truly embrace and practice the principle of self-determination, I contend we are co-participants in Alaska Native communities. We do not enter rural Native communities with our own agendas, but rather we support the positive things Native people are doing on an individual level as well as a community level. Moreover, we do not work alone but alongside Native individuals. By adopting a decolonizing posture, we create room to work within a co-participatory relationship with our Native colleagues—valuing their knowledge, their worldviews, and their contribution to their community.

Participation is essential to development (Bopp and Bopp 2006). If we, as non-Native outsiders, perceive ourselves and assert ourselves as the only participants in community interventions, then we assume an elitist posture that only serves to affirm our egos and not the inherent strengths of Alaska Natives. We must enter Alaska Native communities with the attitude that we are not experts but rather co-participants in a process within which we must work interdependently with Native people and not in arrogant isolation.

Non-Native mental health professionals can provide support toward this vision by supporting the work of behavioral health aides and behavioral health practitioners. Although we may have advanced knowledge of mental health theories, tools, and techniques, we do not possess an understanding of what it is like to be Native nor do we have intimate knowledge of negotiating village life and relating to Native individuals like the village-based professional has. As such, we must respect their knowledge as much or more so than the knowledge we acquired from our college educations. Furthermore, recognizing substantial empirical research demonstrating that paraprofessionals are equally effective helpers when compared to professionals (Durlak 1981; Hattie, Sharpley, and Rogers 1984), Native counselors must be given the respect they deserve. We must not assume that there is a direct correlation between a therapist's training and a therapist's efficacy.

Anything I do on a professional level within a Native village, I strive to do jointly with the village-based BHA/BHP. This includes doing individual psychotherapy sessions together, community workshops together, family sessions together, prevention activities together, meeting with Native agencies together, and interfacing with school personnel together. Village-based personnel possess invaluable knowledge in conducting these activities, and they bring a Native perspective that is absolutely crucial—a perspective I cannot pretend to possess. Without such a Native perspective, a non-Native mental health professional works in cultural isolation. When we exclude village-based personnel, we risk promoting our own ethnocentrism at the expense of empowering Native people and their communities.

Further, it is vital for licensed mental health professionals to not overshadow the work of village-based mental health personnel. I endorse a background presence in Native communities, not interfering with village-based BHAs and BHPs when they take control of situations within their communities.

Additionally, I am cognizant of outside agencies not respecting village-based personnel. In fact, they may attempt to usurp such personnel altogether. We must be ready to not participate in such behavior.

In summary, the BHA/BHP program lies in the foreground of mental health and substance abuse intervention in Native communities. Outside licensed mental health providers may support such interventions but should assume a background and/or co-participatory presence.

4. The Role of the Mental Health Professional Is Multifaceted and Collectively Mindful

If mental health professionals, particularly non-Natives, working in Alaska Native communities adhere rigidly to the positions they trained for in the Lower 48, then their service will be severely limited and short-sighted. We must be careful not to perpetuate the Western model of healthcare that focuses on individualistic values but rather be mindful of the relational fabric that runs through Native communities in a collectivistic spirit.

We must embrace numerous roles, including (but not limited to) prevention advocate, therapist, crisis counselor, friend, consultant, educator, active community member, health aide assistant, and facilitator. Moreover, we must maintain a flexible attitude, such as expecting to work in the evening or making home visits. We must behave in a manner that reinforces behavioral health aides and practitioners promoting wellness in their own people by linking traditional knowledge and practices in the treatment of their clients. This may involve supporting trips with youth to a fish camp in the summer, doing educational talks on the prevention of bullying within the school, or participating in weekly Elder lunches.

Retaining a rigid Western mindset for doing mental health and substance abuse intervention is likely to prevent opportunities for facilitating positive change. Further, it may conflict with and minimize the collectivistic values prevalent in Native communities. We may not want to move in the direction and manner a village pulls us—just like I did not want to "dance" with the wind and the waves on the ocean—but we must be open and receptive to such engagement, although we may harbor some reluctance. Expanding our ways of thinking while performing mental health and substance abuse treatment is needed.

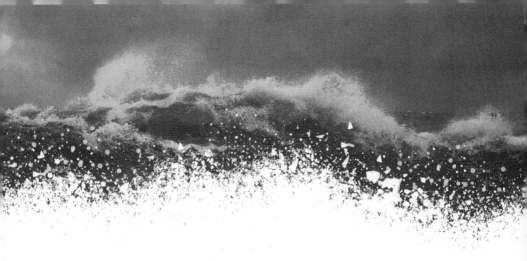

CHAPTER THREE

Cultural Considerations When Working in Alaska Native Communities

Like entering an ocean on an open boat, mental health providers, particularly non-Native ones, have much to consider before beginning work within an Alaska Native community. Being mindful of these issues can cultivate a more culturally sensitive presence in our interactions with Native people and the resources within their communities. Many of the following factors invariably overlap with one another, but I isolate them here to provide more emphasis to their discussion.

Mindset, Transference Issues, and the Strengths of Alaska Native Communities

What is the mindset of a mental health worker bent on working in a rural Alaska Native village? There must be a passion or energy driving them. But, most importantly, this passion must be tempered by an openness toward learning paired with an optimistic spirit.

When I initially came to Nome in late December 1995, I felt privileged to be in such a rural location on Earth. I was fascinated by how well the people of Nome seemed to live, how they cared about their community. I recall watching community volunteers entertain youth on New Year's Eve at the Nome Recreation Center, providing them with healthy activities. I thought, I want to learn how people live here. Not only in Nome but in the outlying Native villages as well. (Little did I know at the time that within two years I would be asked by the Behavioral Health Administration to live and work in a Native community to help support their village-based counseling program.)

We can come to rural Alaska fueled by a sense of adventure and excitement. And there is nothing wrong with taking advantage of programs that benefit us (e.g., the National Health Service Corps, a federal program that repays the student loans of healthcare providers who work in underserved areas). But we must also have a willingness to learn and a passion for working in rural Alaska. Being open to learning is paramount when working within rural Alaska communities. Moreover, our sense of excitement and our willingness to learn must also be reinforced by an attraction toward seeing the good things, the positive things, occurring within Native communities. If we only see the bad, then our behavior and our thoughts are likely to be skewed by such a bias. If a person is compromised at observing the positives in potentially challenging situations, they likely are compromised working in many situations in the world, and probably do not make a good fit for rural Alaska.

Transference issues harbored by non-Native providers must also be considered. As Duran (2006) maintains, non-Native mental health providers may have training in the concept of transference, yet its application to Native peoples is lacking: "there is little mention or training that deals with therapists projecting fantasies of the noble savage or a negative stereotype on the person seeking help" (31). On one end of the transference continuum, non-Native providers may perceive Natives as inferior human beings, while at the other end they may be unrealistically portrayed as holding mystical qualities. Therapeutic work, as a result, can become entangled in a web of projections that hinders the therapeutic relationship. These projections, of course, can also be directed at Native communities.

Our countertransference issues must also be considered. Delving into the vulnerable areas of our clients' lives—Native and/ or non-Native—can be scary, particularly for unseasoned clinicians. What may appear as our clients' avoidance in dealing with traumatic material may in actuality be our own avoidance and reluctance to approach our clients concerning areas of their lives that are unhealed and quite traumatic. When planning trauma work, therapists and clients may unwittingly collude by opting to digress to other issues due to anxiety on both sides about addressing traumatic material.

Alaska Native communities have significant strengths, and these must be at the forefront of awareness for mental health workers. Over twenty years of living and working in the Bering Strait region, I have observed the assets of Native political infrastructure encompassing the Indian Reorganization Act (IRA), Native corporations, and the Indian Child Welfare Act (ICWA). Regarding the latter, I have witnessed ICWA workers' devotion to youth in their community and their fight to ensure that Native children are not unfairly removed from their families and communities. A similar devotion can be seen in Native workers embracing their roles in the BHA Program, as well as the Alaska Federation of Natives (AFN). Native programs advancing economic development in the Bering Strait region are also clearly visible. The tri-owned reindeer herd in Stebbins and St. Michael, for example, has grown significantly since it was established several decades ago. The Kawerak Reindeer Herders Association (RHA), comprised of twenty-one members, assists the development of a self-sustaining reindeer industry in rural Alaska. The Norton Sound Economic Development Corporation (NSEDC), too, is an incredibly successful program providing economic development through education, employment, training, and financial assistance to its fifteen member communities. We must not forget the wisdom of Native Elders and their contribution to their communities, as well as the strong relational ties that run through Native families and their villages. These relational ties are reflected in the rich, spiritual connection Natives have with the land and its natural resources. We must also recognize research contradicting stereotypes of widespread alcohol abuse among Alaska Natives (see, for example, Skewes and Lewis 2016).

Still, there is much talk about the negatives and the many challenges in rural Alaska, and these will be discussed here as well. But mental health providers must not forget about the strengths lest we engage in a downward spiral that contributes to a mindset that is incapable of observing, reinforcing, and demonstrating the values of empowerment in Native communities. This is particularly crucial given optimism's contribution to positive physical and mental health functioning (Conner, DeYoung, and Silvia 2016; Jayawickreme, Forgeard, and Seligman 2012; Kivimaki et al. 2005; Vazquez et al. 2009) and empirical support for its cross-cultural presence (Gallagher, Lopez, and Pressman 2013; Smokowski et al. 2014). Further, optimism is not a static condition but can be fostered and learned (Bates 2015; Lyubomirsky and Layous 2013).

Collective Colonizing Trauma and Specific Traumas on Native Communities

In a Native cemetery in the Bering Strait region lies a prominent tombstone honoring the founder of a fundamentalist religious sect and his accomplishment: "When he arrived in this village there was no Christian. When he died there was no heathen."

On St. Lawrence Island, in the Native community of Gambell, there is an apology letter—framed and hanging in their lodge—from the Presbytery of Yukon. The letter openly acknowledges that through their schools and ministry, the church failed to understand the Natives of Gambell. It specifically states:

we have acted in ways that contributed to the loss of the St. Lawrence Island Yup'ik language, caused confusion about proper use of Native drums and other cultural objects, and caused confusion for some about how to understand their identity in this world. (March 10, 2012)

Colonizing influences by dominant cultures on Native Alaskans have been richly and tragically portrayed in historical literature (see, for example, Michener 1988 and Roesch 1990). Mental health professionals have recognized these influences as significant contributors to the anguish and suffering of many Native people (Duran and Duran 1995). Such influences can be characterized as a form of psychological maltreatment in that Native people were forced to relinquish their own identity in lieu of the dominant culture. Insisting that Natives give up their language, their traditional ceremonies, their cultural practices—all are examples of a concerted attack on the self. This process of devaluing the very substance of Native identity is, in essence, an oppression of the heart, the soul, and the spirit. And it has led to a significant disruption in the development of positive Native self-concept. Alcohol abuse, domestic violence, depression, anxiety, and suicide have been seen as attempts to take control of the internalized turmoil of a sabotaged, defeated, shamed, oppressed sense of Native self (Duran and Duran 1995; Napoleon 1996).

Exacerbating these oppressive forces are additional forms of maltreatment that have torpedoed the Native ego. Child sexual abuse by priests, for example, has been increasingly acknowledged by Native Americans (Middelton-Moz 1999). In their seminal work, *Sex, Priests, and Secret Codes* (2006), Doyle, Sipe, and Wall document the history of silence that has plagued the Catholic Church from the post-Apostolic centuries to the present. They maintain that this secrecy has deterred the church from dealing openly and honestly with the investigation of clerical perpetrators of sexual abuse of children. In the Frontline documentary *The Silence* (2011), Central Yup'ik Natives from the village of St. Michael in the Bering Strait region share their victimization by Father George Endal and Joseph Lundowski, a former Trappist monk and Catholic volunteer recruited by Endal, between 1968 and 1975. In a passionate, honest, and humble manner, Father Bergquist writes in *The Long Dark Winter's Night* (2010) that the Church must first realize its loss. To do so, he suggests that the Church must go through its own stages of grieving to take honest ownership of the sex scandal. With this new acceptance, laden with honesty and humbleness, a new norm for the Church can be achieved. James Carroll (2019), a Catholic priest from 1969 to 1974, maintains that clericalism and its hierarchical power and culture of silence and denial is the foundation of Roman Catholic dysfunction. Carroll, still a devout Catholic, argues that to save the Church, Catholics must detach from the clerical hierarchy and that the priesthood should be abolished.

Patterns of sexual abuse in Aboriginal families and communities in Canada have been viewed as directly related to the sexual abuse committed by the non-Aboriginal staff of their residential boarding schools (Bopp and Bopp 1997). Such abuse, and other harmful effects (e.g., humiliating punishments) of residential boarding schools, spurred the Canadian government to issue a formal apology to its Aboriginal people in January 1998. Giago's *Children Left Behind* (2006) provides a personal account of the abuse of helpless children in one Indian mission boarding school coupled with the history of the government's role and misguided assimilation efforts via mission boarding schools in the lives of Native people. Napoleon's *Yuuyaraq: The Way of the Human Being* (1996) provides another personal account of trauma, loss, and the disruption of familial ties due to the great many deaths that occurred among Native families in Alaska when diseases were introduced into the communities by traders, whalers, and missionaries. I found it emotionally exhausting to read Napoleon's book. For me, it must be read several times to truly assimilate the message of loss and trauma he so concisely captures in the histories of his own Yup'ik people.

Consistent with Napoleon's discussion of how outsiders introduced diseases to Native communities, I digress for a moment to share my being deployed by the United States Public Health Service on March 10, 2020 to provide mental health support during the coronavirus outbreak. Within two weeks of being deployed, I became concerned about my eventual return to the Bering Strait region. I was very much aware of how the Spanish flu pandemic of 1918 decimated many Native communities [e.g., influenza in November of 1918 killed 72 of 80 Native inhabitants in one village] and I did not want to be responsible for introducing the coronavirus to the Bering Strait region. Fortunately, by the time my deployment was finished the governor of Alaska had made it mandatory for all people entering the state from the Lower 48 to undergo a 14-day quarantine in Anchorage; further, the Native communities—including Nome—in the Bering Strait region had also imposed a mandatory 14-day quarantine for all people entering the area from Anchorage. I was reassured that I had an entire month of quarantine during which I received testing for the virus three times with negative results.

Compounding the effects of colonization, many Native communities experience multiple traumatic deaths with great frequency (Brave Heart et al. 2016), leaving layers of unresolved trauma and loss. One day, a Native client who had endured many personal deaths of family members came to me and explained that she had just lost a sister to alcohol; she was adamantly not going to grieve her loss because she had too many other things to focus on, such as her job and her family.

The rate of suicidal deaths among Alaska Natives has been observed to be two to over three times compared to U.S. whites (Day, Provost, and Lanier 2006; Holck, Day, and Provost 2013). In a study conducted by the Alaska State Department of Health and Social Services from 2003 to 2008, Alaska Native men between the ages of twenty and twenty-nine committed suicide at a rate more than thirteen times the national average. Alaska, too, experiences a high death rate due to unintentional injury stemming from factors such as being employed in high-risk jobs (e.g., mining, construction, oil extraction, and fishing); rural areas in particular are subjected to many risk factors, including weather conditions and lack of access to healthcare due to great distances (Alaska Injury Surveillance Report 2011).

Adverse childhood experiences (ACEs) are strong predictors of adult health risks and disease (Danese et. al. 2009). Consistent with these findings, the historical trauma of Native peoples has been seen "as a contributing cause in the development of illnesses such as PTSD, depression and Type 2 diabetes" (Pember 2016). Native historical or intergenerational trauma is conceptualized as having three stages: (1) the dominant culture perpetuates colonial influences on a population; (2) the affected population manifests physical and psychological symptoms; and (3) the initial affected population passes their trauma responses to subsequent generations (Pember 2016). The passing of the effects of unresolved trauma from one generation to another, moreover, may have biological underpinnings—grounded in epigenetics where external or environmental factors modify the activation of genes but not the genetic code sequence of DNA. In a 2008 study, conducted by Moshe Szyf at McGill University in Montreal, the brains of suicide victims were found to have high levels of glucocorticoids, which can alter gene expression. Szyf asserted that genes were switched off in response to events such as abuse during childhood. Additionally, Native researcher Teresa Brockie at the National Institutes of Health suggests that gene methylation is linked to health disparities among Native Americans (Brockie, Heinzelmann, and Gill 2013). She and her colleagues documented that the high rate of ACEs among Native Americans is associated with the methylation of genes that regulate the stress response.

Colonization processes that marginalized and oppressed Native Alaskans have given Native people the message that somehow they are inferior human beings: lacking, subaverage, subhuman, pagan, "heathen." Working with many Alaska Natives, I have heard how they feel ashamed of their culture and their traditions. This is internalized oppression. Duran (2006) characterizes the historical, intergenerational trauma of Native peoples as a spiritual or soul wound: "Manifestation of the internalized soul wound is found in many facets of life, such as domestic violence, suicide, family dysfunction, community dysfunction and violence, institutional violence and dysfunction, tribal/political infighting and violence, spiritual abuse and violence, and epistemic violence" (22–23).

Kotzebue Iñupiat William Hensley (2009), who helped establish the Alaska Federation of Natives (AFN) in 1966, similarly had the realization of the spiritual wound of his people:

> On that wintry beach in Nome, I had an epiphany. For the first time, I suddenly recognized the full extent of the human suffering that had been taking place among our people in the least obvious of places: in our minds and spirits. For the first time, I truly began to understand some profound truths about the nature of identity, culture, and connection and about the systematic measures-especially religious and educational indoctrination-used by nations all over the world to destroy the spirit of the minorities within their borders (201).

Alaska Natives have been marginalized in many other ways. When President Obama met with Alaska Native leaders in September 2015, Native leaders impressed upon him their long history of serving a secondary position in decision-making policies governing Native communities. As one Native leader succinctly stated, there is a need for Natives "to graduate from consultation to collaboration" (*Nome Nugget*, September 17, 2015).

Lack of political power among Alaska Natives and Native Americans has led to detrimental policies being promoted at their expense. In the late twentieth century, for example, forced sterilization and abortions were often performed without the full consent and/or knowledge of Native women and under the ethnocentric pretense that sterilization was in their best interest (Dillingham 1977; Larson 1977; Lawrence 2000; Rutecki 2010; Stern 2005; Temkin-Greener et al. 1981; Torpy 2000; Wagner 1977). In a similar vein of national-al exploitation, the rural Native communities of Alaska have been subject to experimental testing encompassing the military's nuclear, chemical, and biological warfare programs (see www.akaction. org). O'Neill's *The Firecracker Boys* (1994) interweaves H-bombs, Iñupiat Natives, and the roots of the environmental movement in an epic story of Project Chariot. Outspoken Alaskans effectively deterred the Atomic Energy Commission from exploding nuclear bombs intended to create an experimental harbor near Cape Thompson. Still, fresh radioactive fallout from Nevada was brought to and buried in nearby Ogotoruk Valley in 1962 to find out if exploded nuclear bombs would contaminate local drinking water. In the thirty years that followed this experiment, Point Hope residents experienced a high rate of cancer-related deaths. Local Natives pushed for the contaminated site to be excavated and barged away. The federal government appropriated $3 million to subsequently clean up the site (Vandegraft 1993).

One Native Elder shared with me how the high inhalant abuse in her village was directly linked to the seemingly innocuous visit of a White outsider from Anchorage who wanted to teach children about the dangers of inhalants. This individual led workshops in the school. He brought with him a host of household items on which one could get high to warn of the dangers of inhaling them. Upon this person's departure, the village had a dramatic increase in inhalant abuse within its youth, and this trend continues to date.

The aforementioned example of how outsiders can adversely introduce information to a Native community underscores the need for collaborative relationships. When I present on a topic such as suicide awareness in an Alaska Native village, I attempt to do it collaboratively with Natives who know their community. I strive to do community presentations in concert with individuals who can impart their own perspectives and insight.

Global warming has also made an impact in the Arctic. In the early 1990s, residents of Shishmaref, an Iñupiat community in the northern portion of the Bering Strait region, began noticing the sea around their island freezing later each fall and thawing earlier in the spring. This made the island more vulnerable to sea surges and led to the loss of more than 200 feet of shoreline since 1969 (Mele and Victor 2016). In February 2017, Shishmaref residents voted to relocate to a new site on the mainland at an estimated cost of $100 to $200 million, a process expected to take twenty to thirty years, depending on funding (BHA and former mayor Donna Barr, personal communication, 2019).

Changes in weather patterns and poor ice conditions have also impacted Native subsistence. In 2013, for example, a poor walrus harvest experienced by Gambell and Savoonga hunters on St. Lawrence Island led to a Native food shortage, "prompting the State of Alaska to declare an economic disaster, which did very little in terms of alleviating the food shortage" (*Nome Nugget*, July 2014).

In the summer of 2019, the Norton Sound region experienced salmon die-offs in unusually large numbers from villages in eastern Norton Sound to the Nome area. Dead pre-spawned pink salmon—appearing healthy—were found floating in rivers. While salmon die-offs are natural, the numbers were larger than what is normally observed. Higher water temperatures, coupled with a high concentration of fish, were believed to be the cause of the pink salmon die-off (Hovey 2019).

Climate change has not only affected the physical health of some Arctic Natives but has had secondary adverse effects on mental health and well-being as well (Clayton et al. 2017). Several Inuit communities in Canada, closely connected to the land and environment, have experienced significant stress from the need to adapt to the changing climate. Traditions of hunting, trapping, fishing, foraging, and harvesting are being compromised due to climate change. Some reported adverse effects include weakened social networks, increased levels of conflict, increased drug and alcohol use, and reduced self-sufficiency. One member of an Inuit community explained the stress on Native self-identity as: "We are people of the sea ice. If there's no more sea ice, how can we be people of the sea ice?" (Clayton et. al. 2017, 32).

The military presence in Alaska Native communities is an additional trauma that cannot be underestimated. Since the 1940s, Alaska has been an important US military location due to its close proximity to Russia. In the Norton Sound region, for example, "World War II saw a massive expansion of military activities in the region" (Hogan, Christopherson, and Rothe 2006). Due to fears that, after the attack on Pearl Harbor, the Japanese might move north beyond the Aleutian Chain, over 40,000 troops were stationed in the Nome area. In the early 1950s, the fear of a Japanese attack was replaced by the fear of attack by the Soviet Union. National Guard facilities were established in several villages in the Bering Strait region. Many of these sites, now abandoned, still have significant contaminants present. Residents of St. Lawrence Island, for example, are concerned that their high rates of cancer are linked to the pollutants in their land, which they rely upon for subsistence fishing, hunting, and plant gathering. The document *Formerly Used Defense Sites (FUDS) in the Norton Sound Region* provides a comprehensive history of areas in Norton Sound that had a military presence (e.g., White Alice Sites) and the status of their clean-up efforts (https://www.akaction.org/wp-content/uploads/2015/07/Norton_Sound_FUDS_report_2006. pdf).

Culture of Silence

I have heard Native youth share their pain and frustration toward grandparents reluctant to talk about their culture. They talk about how they came to emulate their Elders' silence due to their own feelings of shame toward sharing their own culture. I have also heard from Elders how they keep secret their special gift of intuitively knowing something is amiss, how such shamanistic knowledge is hidden within their communities. Families who have shamanistic histories rarely share such information openly. Community problems such as suicide are also often deferred to a culture of silence in the belief that acknowledging such problems somehow gives them more power.

The process of oppression on a culture encourages silence where its members are reluctant to give voice to the various forms of oppression they have experienced. Often, this reticence breeds symptoms that mask the true underlying pain of oppression: violence toward self and/or others, alcoholism, depression, anxiety, relational problems, interactions with the legal system, and sometimes outright psychosis. This shame-based silence emanates from many oppressive influences, such as the boarding school influence that emphasized assimilation into the White man's world at the expense of the loss of Native language and traditions steeped in dancing, singing, and drumming.

I have observed young adults as well sharing how their own parents were prone to silence, submissiveness, and shame—attributing these traits to how their parents were punished by boarding school teachers for speaking their Native language.

Brazilian educator Paulo Freire[4] introduced the "culture of silence" in his book *Pedagogy of the Oppressed* (1970), which articulates the dynamics that effectively dominate people in colonized countries. This imposed silence is not necessarily an absence of response but rather an inability to critically respond to what has and is taking place in dominated individuals. Often, individuals internalize negative images of themselves and feel disempowered, immersed in hopelessness and a culture of silence. Similar manifestations of this phenomenon are observed in victims of rape and domestic violence.

---

4   I am grateful for the wisdom of Ward Walker, who shared his reverence toward the work of Freire and how he has applied it in his work in Alaska Native communities.

When oppressed people develop a critical consciousness, this sets in motion a synthesis of thought and action where people can reclaim their humanity. Liberation is achieved from within the oppressed, who must come to a critical understanding of reality, which potentially leads to action.

Freire applies this process to the teacher–student relationship, asserting that solutions must not be predetermined by the teacher but must come together during a process of dialogue. That is, the teacher and the student learn from each other.

The theory of dialogic communication came from Martin Buber (1878–1965), a professor of philosophy at Hebrew University who focused on the way humans relate to the world. He believed that when people truly make themselves completely available to others, understanding them, sharing with them without pretense, a bond is created that leaves each person in that interaction enhanced in some way.

Freire described four oppressive forces that undermine dialogic communication: (1) conquest, where the conqueror imposes objectives on the conquered, making the latter an object of possession; (2) division, where the oppressors further weaken the oppressed via repressive methods to maintain their division through various means (e.g., government policies that give the impression of helping but in fact disempower them); (3) manipulation, a fundamental instrument for the preservation of domination; and (4) cultural invasion, where the oppressors impose their own view of the world upon those they dominate and inhibit creativity by curbing their expression.

This lack of critical expression—the inability to identify and articulate the dynamics of oppression—is essential to keep people oppressed. But the voices of Alaska Natives are increasingly being heard. Many Alaska Natives have given form and meaning to their lives in spite of hardship (e.g., Napoleon 1996; Frontline 2008; Walker 2014). I have been privileged, too, to personally hear stories of Alaska Natives fighting for their rights. In the 1970s in one Native school district, a woman shared with me how education services were lacking for her disabled daughter and how she advocated for her child to receive special education after threatening the superintendent with a lawsuit. Today, as a result of her advocacy, this school district now has full special education services accommodating disabled Native children.

Native healers, too, are receiving the recognition and validation they deserve that has supported them and energized them toward positive action: "After generations of silence our traditional healers once hidden, condemned, or misunderstood, are finally reviving the rich history of our peoples to help heal our communities" (Alaska Native Tribal Health Consortium, 2014, p. 105).

A quiet Native man[5] in one Native community came to me in crisis—tears flowing from his tired eyes, looking physically and emotionally exhausted. He explained, rather reluctantly, that he was being abused at his seasonal job. Clearly, the abuse he was experiencing was violence perpetuated by his employer. I thought to myself that an employment lawyer would be eager to take on his case. But I did not share such thoughts, and instead asked him what he was going to do about it. He explained that the abuse had gone on for several months, yet he hesitated to approach his company's human relations director. He went on to say that he had been a "wallflower" all his life, and had difficulty speaking up for himself even when circumstances justified it. He shared how he had learned this behavior from his parents, who were also prone to not speaking their mind, and he attributed it to the abuse they had endured in the boarding schools they had attended in their youth, where they were punished for speaking their Native language and expressing anything that had the flavor of their culture. He added that his father—although quiet in public—was quite angry and controlling within his own home. His father's angry tendencies made my client even more withdrawn and

---

5   Case presentations are disguised to protect the anonymity of individuals. Any similarities to real people are purely unintentional and coincidental.

passive, and these behavioral traits extended into his adulthood after he married and had children of his own.

I talked with this man about how he had the opportunity to end the intergenerational silence that was passed on to him from his parents and possibly his parents' parents. More importantly, he could be a role model to his young children on how not to be silent when silence only served to extend suffering. He considered the words we had exchanged. Toward the end of our session, he abruptly stood up and said firmly, "I know what to do." In subsequent sessions, this client arrived with improved affect, carrying himself with increased self-confidence, sharing the aftermath of making a report of abuse to his HR director, and also exploring other options such as hiring an attorney.

Collectivism

The villages I have worked with in the Bering Strait region are strongly relational and collectivistic. Individuals perceive themselves as part of a whole: family, tribe, or community. Relationships within family, tribe, and community carry high significance. Even when there is feuding among families, these conflicts become secondary in times of loss and tragedy: people drop their disagreements and come together to support those in need.

Wellness is often defined as being grounded in traditional tribal lifestyle and connected to community and nature. The importance of social functioning and connection to nature has been empirically supported in the perceptions of wellness among the Yup'ik in the Yukon-Kuskokwim Delta (Wolsko et al. 2006). The importance of being connected to extended kinship family structure in Alaska Native adolescents living in rural remote communities has also received support (Fok, Allen, and Henry 2014).

To simply perceive Alaska Natives as collectivistic, however, can present as a stereotype, and potentially undermine an understanding of the complexities of life currently confronting Alaska Natives. I have observed how, in some communities that are more bicultural (i.e., Natives who are capable and comfortable living in their traditional world as well as the Western world), individualism and collectivism are not considered polar opposites but rather coexist dynamically. Relationships and community still carry a high degree of importance, but becoming autonomous and functional as an adult is also perceived as an essential expectation. Parents push their children to go to college or acquire a skill at a vocational school. Native individuals, too, may exhibit both traits of collectivism and individualism depending on their specific context. For example, a Native may be assertive, competitive, and self-efficient at work but submissive to parents and uphold traditional familial views within their home. The dynamic coexistence of individualism and collectivism in other cultures has been observed (see, for example, Tamis-LeMonda et al., 2008). As the social, political, and economic pressures of acculturation impinge on their communities, Alaska Native youth must reconcile maintaining the relatedness of their traditional culture versus pursuing the goal of autonomy in the Western world.

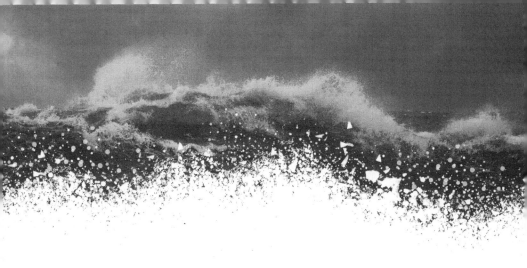

CHAPTER FOUR

Therapy Considerations

Relational-Cultural Theory

The variables of marginalization, internalized oppression, shame, disempowerment, and the value of relatedness beg for a theory for performing mental health work with Alaska Natives. I propose that relational-cultural theory best captures the dynamics that provide a sound framework for mental health therapy with Alaska Natives.

Relational-cultural theory, and by extension, relational-cultural therapy (RCT), comes from the work of Jean Baker Miller, MD, and is often aligned with the feminist movement in psychology in the 1970s. In *Toward a New Psychology of Women*, Miller (1976) delineates the dynamics of dominance and subordination in the psychology of women. The theory was further developed by women psychologists at the Stone Center at Wellesley College, including Judith V. Jordan, Janet Surrey, and Irene Stiver. One of its core tenets is to delineate oppressive systems and give voice to marginalized populations, both men and women. RCT addresses many social injustices that disempower and disrupt human connection at both the individual and societal level. It speaks to all human beings wherever sociocultural forces misunderstand, invalidate, exclude, humiliate, or injure a person, leading to pervasive disconnection in human relationships characterized by self-blame, feelings of immobilization, and isolation (Jordan 2010). The experiences of disconnection are perceived as contributing to a state of human suffering, manifesting in many forms. Mutual growth-fostering relationships are seen as a vital force for healthy reconnection and increased prosocial functioning. The emphasis on a *mutual* process of engagement is consistent with Freire's (1970) dialogic process of communication.

Relational-Cultural Therapy and Multicultural Care

If we assume that Alaska Natives experience various forms of disempowerment and disconnection, then interventions that empower them and serve to reconnect them in many ways would form the core for working with them. I contend that RCT is applicable to mental health professionals working in rural Alaska Native communities. RCT, which emerged as the fourth wave of theories of psychotherapy, is grounded in feminist and multicultural theories (Frew and Spiegler 2008). Reflecting on my experience on the ocean, I became disconnected when I attempted to navigate in directions that only made matters worse and threatened my life. It was only when I became mindful of myself, and attuned to the behavior of the Bering Sea, that I could make changes that allowed me and the ocean to flow rhythmically, to be engaged in a mutual exchange that offered maximum energy and connection. In the same manner, RCT acknowledges the importance of the therapeutic relationship and a mutual engagement between therapist and client. When therapists are authentic, responsive, and offer a nondefensive presence with their client, the therapeutic relationship becomes a rich source for positive change (Jordan 2010).

Given the lack of research on Natives in Alaska and the Lower 48, is any research on therapy applicable toward our work with Alaska Natives? As one Yup'ik professional commented, we can take what is good from both worlds: Native and Western culture as well. It is prudent, therefore, to peruse the literature on which components of psychotherapy promote positive outcome. In the seminal work by the American Psychological Association Division 29 task force (Norcross 2001, 2002), elements of effective therapy relationships and effective methods used to tailor individual therapy were identified in a series of meta-analyses.

The most important predictor of positive outcome in psychotherapy has nothing to do with the therapy itself. Events outside of therapy (e.g., ego strength, social support) were found to account for 40 percent of positive outcomes. Of the 60 percent that we as helpers can influence, 30 percent is contingent upon the development and maintenance of a good therapeutic relationship (e.g., empathy, warmth, and encouragement of risk-taking). The remaining 30 percent is split equally between positive expectancy (also called "hope" or "placebo") and techniques /models. One might argue at this point that our techniques and methods of psychotherapy, grounded in evidence-based practice, do not compare to the therapeutic impact of the therapy relationship.

There is a good argument, too, that the relational component in positive therapy outcome is even greater than 30 percent. The process of developing expectancy/hope/placebo, for example, can be viewed as having a relational function; if so, the degree we can influence positive outcomes for our clients rises even more. I must add that I find it difficult to separate employing methods and techniques of therapy with the therapeutic relationship because there is a degree of trust, faith, and belief—due to the relationship itself—that is embedded in the process of employing techniques. For example, I use eye movement desensitization reprocessing (EMDR) with some

Native clients with complex trauma, and I always fall back on my "clinical seat" when something does not feel right. If I sense that a client is not ready for EMDR, I back up and pay attention to that— engaging the client in a mutual dialogue rather than simply doing EMDR without regard for the client's readiness.

The compelling body of research gleaned from the APA task force identified three robust relational elements: empathy, alliance, and goal consensus and collaboration.

1. Empathy

Empathy is linked to outcome because it serves a positive relationship function and facilitates a corrective emotional experience, promotes exploration and meaning creation, and supports clients' active healing.

In one study (Bachelor 1988), 44 percent of clients valued a cognitive form of empathic response, 30 percent an affective form of empathy, and 26 percent a nurturing and disclosing empathic response. The bottom line: no single empathic response exists. Clients respond according to their own unique needs, and it is important to convey empathy to all clients in all forms of psychotherapy.

2. Alliance

Alliance refers to the quality and strength of the collaborative relationship between client and therapist. Interestingly, the positive impact of the alliance is not restricted to psychotherapy: several studies have supported this within prescribing physician–patient relationships.

Further, one central force that I have consistently found to be vital to promoting a good therapeutic alliance is being a good listener. I strongly believe that having good listening skills, being able to be quiet with a client coupled with an attentive ear, is paramount for good psychotherapy.

Some recommended clinical practices, stemming from the element of alliance, are:

- Develop a strong alliance early in treatment, probably within three to five sessions. If the alliance has not solidified by the fifth session, then the probability for success is jeopardized.
- Recognize that the alliance is harder to establish with clients who are more disturbed, delinquent, homeless, drug-abusing, fearful, anxious, dismissive, or preoccupied.
- Foster a stronger alliance by using communication skills, empathy, and openness.
- Strive to reach consensus on goals and respective tasks, which contributes to alliance formation and then to treatment success.
- Emphasize, particularly in the initial sessions, the relational bond, the special sense of understanding, safety, and trust.

3. Goal Consensus and Collaboration

Collaborative therapists attend verbally to clients' problems. They address topics of importance to clients. Collaborative therapists resonate to client attribution of blame regarding their problems. In short, the therapist and client journey together toward a mutual destination.

I contend that these three elements are culturally applicable to Alaska Natives because they speak to the relationship that I have found essential when working with Alaska Natives—and, for that matter, all clients. Being empathic, respectful, connected, and genuine has been found to be expected among American Indians and other multicultural clients (Trimble et al. 1996; Comas-Diaz 2012). Comas-Diaz (2012) refers to multicultural individuals as "culturally different individuals and/or people of color (4)." These elements are particularly important in the context of working with Alaska Natives because of their histories laden with relationships that have left them disempowered, invalidated, dismissed, and exploited. Further, the symptoms that often come to the forefront when beginning psychotherapy mask the damaged relational images Native clients hold. Mental health professionals working in rural Alaska Native communities must be sensitive to the unseen damaged relationships held in the souls of our clients lest we lose perspective and simply focus on the presenting symptoms (e.g., alcoholism, abuse, anxiety, depression, suicidal ideation, anger, violence). In the context of a caring therapeutic relationship, the deep hurt our clients hold can be healed and the problems they present with can be worked on. We may not work in the manner of a Native mental health professional (e.g., Duran 2006), but our presence, our attunement to the therapeutic relationship, can impart a corrective emotional experience that also has positive biologic underpinnings.

Siegel (2010) talks of the synthesis of psychotherapy and neuroscience. He maintains that the therapist's presence and manner of connecting with the client are crucial factors contributing to healing. He states that "our innate temperament and our experiences in attachment and peer relationships together mold our personality" (163). Individuals who exhibit insecure attachment and lead a rigid life have impaired neural integration. The goal of therapy, then, is integration, and this can be achieved through a caring therapeutic relationship. Further, a person does not lose the personality type they have developed; rather, "it seems to move to a more adaptive, flexible, and coherent flow" (163). Individuals who are anxious, for example, are able to step back and laugh at their tendencies toward worrying compared to previously being immersed without any awareness of this trait. When there is neural integration, then, people become more adaptive and harmonious in their functioning.

Mindfulness, Siegel maintains, invites neural integration. Consistent with RCT, this is a mutual process: therapists must first be mindful of their own personalities and their own ability to be fully present. This is a daily process, not an end product: I may be mindful one moment and then lost in the chaos of thinking about the things I need to do later on. Cultivating presence and being mindful as a therapist provides the context, the foundation, for cultivating mindfulness in clients, and we must continually work on being in the moment.

I have found Siegel's acronym PART useful when I am doing therapy since it helps keep me in the moment and connected with my client. Presence (P) imparts being open, flexible, and receptive not only to our own internal state but that of the client before us. Attunement (A) refers to being keenly aware of another's feelings, thoughts, and nonverbal behavioral patterns that may show insight into the person's internal state. Siegel states: "When others sense our attunement with them, they experience 'feeling felt' by us" (34). Resonance (R) involves the connection of the therapist and the client into one whole temporarily, where both are changed as a result of attunement to each other. For example, Siegel offers the example of placing his hand on his heart when he feels the sadness of a client's story. Authentic experience helps clients know that we resonate with their feelings and "enables them to 'feel felt'" (57). Trust (T) is achieved when as therapists we practice presence, attunement, and resonance. Clients feel safe and secure when trust becomes established—enveloped in a healing love without fear.

I recall working with a bright five-year-old boy who was very good at manipulating his mother. I must admit, sometimes I was thrown off by the things he did. For example, his mother once called me in a distraught state—explaining that she had taken her son to the dentist after he had promised to cooperate with getting his teeth clean; once he was there, he refused to open his mouth and his appointment was subsequently terminated. This had occurred several times. The mother put me on the spot and asked me what to do to get her son's teeth cleaned. I thought about this for a while and then told the mother: "Tell Ben that he doesn't have to go to the dentist if he doesn't want to, that you respect the choice he is making to not cooperate with the dentist and get his teeth cleaned. Tell him, 'However, as a caring mother, who does not want your teeth to rot and get cavities, I too must make a choice. So, if you choose to not get your teeth cleaned by the dentist, then I—as a caring mother— must stop buying you drinks that have sugar in them.'" Ben, who was very fond of juices that contained sugar, quickly changed his mind, and opening his mouth at the dentist became a nonissue.

In my work with Ben, however, I found that simply talking to him about the poor choices he was making was not a method for connecting. Like my ocean experience, where I changed navigational tactics, I also changed therapeutic strategies with this boy when I took him into the playroom. There, our interaction eventually led to our wrestling with each other on the mat in the room. At one point, I asked myself, What the hell am I doing? Is this therapy? But I continued nevertheless, because intuitively the activity of physical contact with Ben felt right. He enjoyed our interaction immensely. For the first time, I felt connected with him, and I am sure he also felt connected with me. Through the medium of wrestling I was able to establish a sound therapeutic relationship to the extent that my talking to him about the behavioral choices he was making, and how it contributed to making his mother miserable (and himself as well, since he suffered consequences such as loss of privileges), was a more meaningful intervention. In retrospect, I intuitively engaged in PART: wrestling provided an intense physical presence for this boy; we became acutely attuned to each other; we resonated with each other; and all this contributed to a deep sense of trust and respect to the extent that a working therapeutic relationship was formed. Had I simply sat with him and talked about the poor choices he was making, I would have lost vital relational elements essential for working with him.

Being mindful and responsive to the therapeutic relationship and disconnections therein is a hallmark of RCT. Siegel's book discusses how to enhance mindfulness skills, but there are of course many other resources that teach these skills (e.g., Burdick 2013). I have found that being mindful begins with adequate breathing. Without adequate breathing, being in the moment with oneself and another is difficult. We must first be grounded in order to connect with others. When we are grounded, filled with adequate amounts of oxygen to nourish our bodies, our senses become open to the world, and possibilities for connecting with it increase.

Siegel's concept of resonance is similar to Comas-Diaz's (2012) multicultural concepts of affective attunement and cultural resonance. She emphasizes the importance, when working with culturally different clients and/or people of color, for therapists to place themselves in a "client's cultural shoes while acknowledging differences and similarities between the two of you" (140). This process of affective attunement immerses the therapist in the client's internal world. Empathic understanding and cultural responsiveness, which is the core of healing, emerges from this. When therapists demonstrate cultural empathy, they mitigate the negative effects of cultural disconnection and thereby empower their clients through this reconnection. Further, when therapists understand their clients through clinical skill, cultural competence, and intuition, cultural resonance occurs, which "promotes a convergence between you, the clinician, and your multicultural client" (Comas-Diaz 2012). Comas-Diaz acknowledges cognitive and affective empathy but also adds the importance of intuition: a preconscious nonverbal communication that facilitates a client's feelings of others. Anthropologist Joan Koss-Chioino (2006) coined the term *radical empathy*, which speaks of a type of intuitive relatedness where intra- and inter-individual differences converge into one field of feeling. Interestingly, intuition in psychotherapy can be enhanced if a therapist is open to it and is able to quiet the mind and facilitate a sense of affectual connection to clients without engaging in premature cognitive analysis (Dodge Rea 2001). Comas-Diaz (2012) contends that "when you integrate cognitive, affective, cultural, and radical empathy into your multicultural work, you enhance your multicultural clinical presence" (141).

Psychotherapy with Alaska Natives

There is much literature on counseling services for Native Americans in the Lower 48 (Trimble 2010), yet very little related to counseling Alaska Natives (Hays 2006). Reimer's work (1999) among the Iñupiat focuses on the importance of understanding a Native client's perspective of personal wellness. Hays (2006) provides clinical material illustrating the application of cognitive therapy on Alaska Natives. In my own work (Droby 2000), I identify a strengths-oriented perspective among Alaska Natives and the importance of being sensitive to historical trauma without imposing agendas. Motivational interviewing and the stages of change approach have also been advocated with Alaska Natives—emphasizing the components of listening, learning, respect, and being mindful of Native values and culture (Tomlin et al. 2014).

My working model for performing psychotherapy with Alaska Natives embraces four elements, which I refer to as the 4Rs: relationship; self-regulation skills; reprocessing trauma; and reinforcing a client's work and progress in the context of historical trauma. The first three elements have been identified by Gentry (2014) in his work with traumatized individuals, while the fourth factor is one that I have added from my own work with Alaska Natives.

The 4Rs are grounded in data I took from ten random clients (five female, five male) that sensitized me to the trauma they have suffered: 70 percent of my clients had four or more adverse childhood experiences, compared to the ACE study's 17 percent. This also exceeds the 23.2 percent of Alaska adults who had four or more adverse childhood experiences (2014–2015 Alaska BRFSS,

Section of Chronic Disease Prevention and Health Promotion, Alaska Division of Public Health, and Centers for Disease Control and Prevention; *Behavioral Risk Factor Surveillance System Survey ACE Module Data, 2010*). Additionally, all seven clients who had four or more adverse childhood experiences struggled with symptoms of post-traumatic stress disorder, anxiety, and/or depression comorbid with substance abuse, including alcohol and cannabis. Although I must be careful not to generalize these findings to Native communities due to small size and biased sample (i.e., outpatient population), I believe I can strongly generalize them to my overall clinical caseload. Clearly, the clients I work with have been significantly stressed, significantly traumatized. And the concomitant problems correlating with such trauma are strikingly familiar to the problems the ACE study discovered. Therefore, I recognize a need for an approach that stems from the field of traumatology, although there are nuances that will be discussed here.

Therapeutic Relationship

With research on neuroplasticity demonstrating how human interactions change our brain functioning (Siegel 1999 and 2010), the importance of the therapeutic relationship should never be underestimated or minimized. RCT practitioners refer to these corrective experiences as *growth-fostering relationships* (Jordan 2010). Given the legacy of outsiders who have marginalized people such as Alaska Natives, we do not want to add our names to such a list. Research has found that people who are excluded or marginalized register their hurt in the same area of the brain as physical pain (Eisenberger, Lieberman, and Williams 2003; Eisenberger 2012). Such social injustice and its emotional and biological sequela support RCT's focus on the therapeutic relationship, since social connection is seen as a constant need throughout a person's life. Given the relational ties of many Alaska Natives, and the trauma that has disrupted such ties, nurturing this social connection in the context of a therapeutic relationship is prudent. The importance of a strong relational foundation in the context of counseling with American Indians and Alaska Natives has been recognized (Reimer 1999; Thomason 2011; Trimble 2010). I am often amazed by the fact that many of my Native clients have not had the opportunity to share their negative life experiences with other human beings. This is often due to a level of mistrust toward others in a Native community. The fear of confidential, sensitive personal information being made public leads to repressing and suppressing emotional pain, keeping it within a culture of silence. Hence, a therapeutic confidential relationship offers the opportunity for connecting with another human being without the fear of being shamed and/or losing face and self-worth.

In my two decades of working with Alaska Natives, an integral piece of my mental health work has always centered on the therapeutic relationship. Having a sound therapeutic alliance, composed of mutual respect, genuineness, collaboration, and cultural sensitivity, is the core of any work I do with Alaska Natives. This seems like a no-brainer. Yet in our era that emphasizes evidence-based practices, the therapeutic relationship can be lost, overlooked, minimized, or forgotten in our rush to implement techniques and methods (see, for example, Norcross 2001). For me, practice-based evidence points to the importance of the therapeutic alliance governing anything I do in the realm of Alaska Native mental health work. Some feedback my Native clients have given me regarding the benefits of individual psychotherapy include: "Talking through life's traumas and stresses and *being heard*"; "Helped me feel like I mattered"; "Makes me feel better overall"; and "Helped me have a better mindset on my life."

Hartman and Zimberoff (2004) articulate a comprehensive analysis of corrective emotional experiences in the therapeutic process that capture three primary existential themes:

1. Building ego strength through release of shame and reclaiming worthiness;

2. Building agency through release of helplessness and re-claiming personal power; and
3. Building authenticity through the release of dissoci-ation and identification and reclaiming self-reflective identity (6).

A middle-aged woman came to me in crisis, tearful and distraught, sharing with me how on a recent visit to her brother's home he ig-nored her—electing to pay attention to her adult daughter while feigning complete unawareness to her presence. "I was so hurt," she cried. "I feel like I'm going crazy. How could he behave that way to me? Why does it hurt me so badly?"

Together we explored what we had worked on in her therapy, particularly her relationships with family members. We reviewed the theme of empathetic failures in her childhood—negative relational images of significant people in her life who invalidated her, leaving her with feelings of helplessness, unworthiness, and shame. She un-derstood that the flavor of her interaction (or lack of) with her broth-er was the same: being unnoticed, not cared for, not considered a person of any importance. Her visit with her brother triggered over-whelming residual childhood feelings, and she became devastated.

The client became calmer as she came to understand what she had experienced, knowing that she was not going crazy. We worked on how she could be mindful when she might become similarly trig-gered in the future. I used the "inner child" template to help her un-derstand how there was still a hurt little girl within her who longed to be validated, cared for, and loved. She understood that, realistical-ly, such dependency needs would not be met by her brother or oth-er family members, but that there were other supportive people in her life she could turn to. Moreover, we addressed how she needed to validate herself, acknowledge that inner child, and work on ways to empower herself cognitively as well as behaviorally.

An emotionally present therapist who is responsive to address-ing a client's relational failures can serve as a corrective emotional experience that can be empowering on many levels. For example, many Alaska Natives who have been sexually abused have lost memories of their childhood. These memories become further masked by alcoholism and other addictions. One client whose sobriety was supported in therapy slowly began retrieving memories from his past laden with horrendous abuse as a boy. In his sobriety, the haziness of his past faded and his childhood became clearer. In the context of the therapeutic relationship, he reclaimed personal power that had hindered his ability to be a functional member of society.

Self-Regulation

Self-regulation is "the intentional and conscious process of monitoring and relaxing one's body while in the context of a perceived threat, preventing the sympathetic nervous system (SNS) from achieving dominance" (Baranowsky and Gentry 2015, 164). It is not simply learning how to relax but learning how to assert such relaxation skills when faced with perceived dangers.

Having a sound therapeutic alliance enables me to role model and teach self-regulation methods to my Native clients. One caveat I adhere to: do not impose these techniques without the mutual engagement of clients. We must first practice "being" with our clients rather than "doing," without imposing agendas, before we engage them in possible methods they might embrace for dealing with stress. I am reminded of my experience on the ocean: when I attempted to impose my agenda for reaching land, it only made matters worse; I had to attend to the relationship with the ocean, the wind, and the waves before I could negotiate a plan to safely return to land. Further, I do not engage my clients in any self-regulation techniques I do not personally use myself. That is, I do not ask a client to do something I do not do myself.

Many of my clients struggle with substance abuse problems that are comorbid with features of or outright full-blown post-traumatic stress disorder. (I will discuss this in more depth in the next section.)

These comorbidities are consistent with the literature (Breslau, Davis, and Schultz 2003; Jacobsen, Southwick, and Kosten 2001; Ouimette, Brown, and Najavits 1998). Regulating affect, therefore, is an issue with many clients, and smoking cannabis and/or drinking alcohol offers temporary relief to their basic self-regulatory deficits. With the practice of self-regulation methods in lieu of using substances such as cannabis and/or alcohol, my Native clients have reported decreased cravings for substance use. Again, however, I must emphasize that before self-regulation methods are followed, we must be mindful of having our Native clients engaged in the therapeutic alliance. In their review of what works in substance abuse and dependence treatment, Mee-Lee (2010) and his colleagues found that "the therapeutic relationship contributes 5 to 10 times more to outcome than the model or approach used" (400). Further, "research makes clear that client engagement is the single best predictor of outcome" (400) and that the best way to improve retention and outcome "is to attend to clients' experience of progress and the therapeutic relationship early in treatment" (401).

Once a therapeutic alliance is established, I ask clients if learning a method to regulate their affect to reduce stress would be beneficial to them. Once they embrace the idea of learning self-regulation techniques, I engage them in the method of diaphragmatic breathing in combination with visual imagery. I have found that using these techniques in combination, rather than isolation, produces a more rapid shift to a parasympathetic state of relaxation. (I have demonstrated this productive combination through the use of biofeedback equipment.) Many Native clients also resonate with the use of an Action Plan (Fig. 1), illustrating the dynamic relationship (see, for example, Masters et al. 1987) between feelings (affect), thoughts (cognitions), and doing choices (behavior). I often provide clients with the illustration in Figure 1 to help guide them when they become emotionally triggered by an event so they can identify the negative thinking and doing choices they have made historically. Conversely, they can consider alternative thinking and doing choices that are more positive when experiencing stress to affect the mind-body interrelationship. Further, identifying the triggers that often lead to stress in a client's life is important. Identifying triggers and developing ways to negotiate the accompanying feelings in a cognitive and behavioral manner has been meaningful to many of my Native clients. All of the aforementioned data gleaned from a client can be conveniently illustrated so that clients can take home a copy for personal reference.

A client I worked with initially resisted doing diaphragmatic breathing since her stomach muscles were in pain; however, with several more attempts she suddenly experienced her stomach relaxing. Moreover, her mood became brighter, and she reported sensations of calm that she had never experienced before. This highlights the importance of teaching clients who have significant trauma histories relaxation techniques that reduce sympathetic nervous system activation. Simply learning how to relax when facing sympathetic arousal can be a vital therapeutic intervention even before the work of reprocessing traumatic memories begins. Moving slowly is also important, since some trauma victims may experience relaxation as a frightening phenomenon. I recall working with one individual with a significant trauma history. As she performed diaphragmatic breathing, she became tearful and a terrified look came over her face. She reported that relaxing felt like losing personal, inner control. Thus, we must be mindful that some ways victims of trauma have coped with their pain—although possibly appearing maladaptive on the surface—have allowed them to survive and cope with such pain.

Emotional freedom technique (EFT) offers another possible medium for relieving stress. Flint, Lammers, and Mitnick (2006) outline this easy, teachable technique, employing a self-empowering affirmation statement, the acupressure point sequence, and the nine-gamut tapping sequence, which some of my Native clients have embraced. (Other references include Craig 2011 and Rogers and Bloom 2019.) Emotional freedom technique is also consistent with the triad presented in Figure 1 in that it is a behavioral choice for

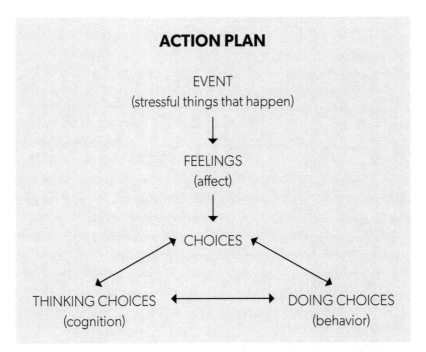

Figure 1. The dynamic relationship between feelings, thoughts, and behavior.

managing stress but also reinforces positive self-affirmations. One Native client who initially implemented this method on herself reported great relief from stress during her day when she used it to help relieve a headache. Further, it had a generalizing effect on relieving stress with other issues in her life.

It should be emphasized that EFT is simply one choice for clients to consider when enhancing self-regulation of their emotional functioning. One study (Waite and Holder 2003) proposed that systematic desensitization and distraction may be the factors contributing to EFT's apparent effectiveness rather than its acupressure point tapping. Still, other studies (Feinstein 2018; Sebastian and Nelms 2017) support its acupoint-based energy psychology protocol for relieving a wide variety of issues, including anxiety and PTSD. Regardless, it is the client who chooses the course to promote self-regulation.

Reprocessing Trauma

In my two decades of working with Alaska Natives in the Bering Strait region and Norton Sound, I have observed that the history of trauma on their culture has been incredibly significant and impactful. Consistent with that history, throughout the body of my clinical caseload, there has been a central vein of traumatization. Unhealed trauma and unresolved inner conflict constitute the common clinical equation. Such symptoms are often masked by alcoholism and/or other drug addictions, suicidal behavior, and violence toward self and/or others. Often, people have difficulty giving "voice" to their inner unhealed pain. People avoid moving to that pain, and such avoidance often leads to self-destructive symptoms.

I habitually use the ACE questionnaire to quickly quantify a client's childhood experiences of abuse and neglect. I prefer using the ACE questionnaire offered by the Indian Health Service.[6] Unlike the standard ACE questionnaire, the IHS questionnaire allows the client to measure to what degree their experience of an adverse childhood experience was on a scale of 0 (not at all) to 10 (very much) when that ACE occurred. It also has a section for the clients to give a current score of how much the same experience bothers them to date. The latter scores are useful since they provide potential indicators of what trauma experiences clients might need and want to work on. I consider the latter scores more important since over time some people can learn to recover from initial traumas they experience. That is, I am not looking at the number of ACEs but rather an individual's current reaction to them; this underscores the importance of recognizing resiliency in the human condition. (Note: I typically administer the ACE questionnaire after a therapeutic alliance has been established, since administering it in the first meeting with a client can be intrusive and potentially render data inaccurate.)

---

6   https://www.ihs.gov/california/tasks/sites/default/assets/File/BP2015-ACESQuestionnaire.pdf

Habitual gathering of ACE data on our mental health clients lends understanding of the depth of adverse trauma experiences our clients may have been exposed to. As mentioned previously, I randomly selected ten clients I work with in the Bering Strait region and Norton Sound. Of these, seven had four or more adverse childhood experiences. In the ACE study, 17 percent of subjects had four or more adverse childhood experiences. Further, the ACE study found that people who had four or more adverse childhood experiences, compared to those who had experienced none, had:

- A four- to twelve-fold increase in health risks for alcoholism, drug abuse, depression, and suicide attempts;
- A two- to four-fold increase in smoking and poor self-rated health;
- A history of greater than or equal to fifty sexual partners and prone to sexually transmitted disease; and
- A 1.4- to 1.6-fold increase in physical inactivity and severe obesity (Felitti et al. 1998).

My clients have had similar problems: substance abuse, anxiety and depression, post-traumatic stress disorder, suicidality, among others.

I have used eye movement desensitization and reprocessing (EMDR) for those clients motivated to reprocess past trauma. I have also employed cognitive-behavioral therapy (CBT). Another promising therapeutic approach I have found for addressing trauma among Alaska Natives (and, for that matter, anyone who is suffering from past unresolved trauma) comes from the field of traumatology. Narrative exposure therapy (NET) is a trauma-informed treatment for survivors of multiple and complex traumas. Briefly, the therapeutic elements of NET involve clients providing a narrative of their traumatic experiences while re-experiencing the emotions associated with the events. This is done repeatedly over several sessions until the client loses their emotional sympathetic nervous system response, leading to remission of PTSD symptoms. Originally developed for use in low-income settings, empirical evidence supports narrative exposure therapy application to traumatized individuals in high-income settings as well. Evidence supports NET as an effective treatment for adults with PTSD as well as children who have been traumatized by conflict and organized violence (Robjant and Fazel 2010). Narrative exposure therapy has been found to be effective along with other tools for treating clients with PTSD such as EMDR and EFT (Gentry 2014). There is also support for the use of trauma-focused exposure therapy in the treatment of co-occurring PTSD and substance use disorders (Baschnagel, Coffey, and Rash 2006).

While there are variations to administering NET, I prefer Gentry's 5-Narrative CBT Model (2014) because it is easy to use, highly structured, and supportive to individuals dealing with unresolved trauma and/or loss. Other resources are available for learning this method (see Baranowsky and Gentry 2015; Gentry 2016). Further, NET stresses the importance of having a supportive therapeutic relationship consisting of empathic understanding, active listening, congruency, and unconditional positive regard—therapist traits recognized as essential when working with Alaska Natives. It recognizes Herman's (1992) Tri-Phasic Model and the importance of providing clients with a battery of self-soothing, grounding techniques when being intruded upon by traumatic memories. This method can be easily taught to mental health providers without going through more complicated, expensive training such as that involved with EMDR, although certainly training is needed to ensure its proper implementation. Listening to a client's narrative of pain and suffering has always been a common denominator in the context of counseling. Narrative exposure therapy, however, offers a more structured medium within which to allow clients to successfully make sense of their suffering—past and present—and to learn how to self-regulate their emotions so that the sympathetic nervous system is not so highly activated to the degree of disrupting daily functioning. Further, it is consistent with Napoleon's (1996) support for talking circles and the belief that the road to health for Alaska Natives involves giving voice to their feelings, experiences, and thoughts within the safety of a supportive audience.

I have some precautions, however, when using NET and other trauma-informed treatments such as EMDR and CBT with Native clients:

- Reprocessing trauma with trauma-informed techniques should not take precedence over having a solid therapeutic alliance. I am careful when implementing these methods, since the motivation for doing so must rest with my client and not only myself. If my motivation exceeds that of my client, then I risk imposing an agenda that does not fit with my client. In this manner, I risk damaging the therapeutic relationship, and perhaps having my client leave therapy prematurely.
- Not all Native clients will want to engage in reprocessing their trauma repeatedly through trauma-informed techniques such as EMDR, NET, and CBT. This should be respected. Some clients may engage in a trauma-informed method one time and choose to stop. The bottom line: reprocessing trauma in a manualized, mechanical manner can be distracting to the therapeutic alliance. In this way, it can disrupt the natural "flow" with clients in a Native community who expect a human interaction with their mental health provider rather than being put through a series of exercises that are intended to reprocess their trauma. That is, without first connecting with a client, and being emotionally attuned to their needs, a mental health provider implementing these methods risks losing their client by imposing an agenda that the client simply does not embrace.
- Some Native clients do not want to reprocess their trauma via structured trauma-informed techniques; it is simply too

anxiety-provoking. Rather, they prefer to narrate their trauma within the context of the therapy relationship. This preference also needs to be respected. I am careful not to cast judgment on whether a client pursues exposure therapy. I am careful not to label such clients as "treatment resistant" or "in denial" or "avoiding."

In short, the 4Rs should not be followed mechanically. Rather, the four elements are potential avenues within the therapeutic process that are aligned with the wind and the waves. I go with what is given. I may offer some avenues or methods for a client to pursue, but in the end I respect their choices for managing and coping with their trauma.

Regarding reprocessing trauma, I have had Native clients who poorly tolerated exposure-based narratives. This is not new in the field of traumatology (see, for example, Foa et al. 2002; Hembree et al. 2003). I am acutely reminded of the wisdom of Duncan, Hubble, and Miller (1997), who, working with difficult cases involving veterans, maintain that our difficult clients must be viewed as human beings first rather than a diagnostic category or a "treatment resistant" case (48).

Duncan et al. (1997) offer the following guidelines, which constitute important reminders to me for maintaining trust in my clients and an uncompromised faith in the therapeutic alliance:

1. *The client is the hero in the "drama" of therapy.* There are no great therapists, only great clients and therapists working together.
2. *Therapy is not done to a client.* It is an interpersonal exchange (event) in which emphasis is placed foremost on the quality of the client's participation.
3. *Interventions are not the "deal" in therapy.* Interventions are extensions of the therapeutic alliance and cannot be separated from the relationship in which they occur.

4. *The therapist suggests, the client chooses.* The therapist offers explanations, theories, or intervention approaches as suggestions for the client to consider and then accept, modify, or discard (49).

Again, I always give clients the freedom to choose whether to engage in trauma-informed methods or simply fall back on emphasizing the therapeutic alliance using active listening, empathy, and cultural attunement, while being mindful of reinforcing a client's self-regulatory skills. This is not avoidance but rather reinforcing the relational component when working with Alaska Natives and their self-regulation skills. I would rather have a client choose not to do a form of trauma-informed therapy and still attend their therapy appointment instead of not showing up for therapy and terminating treatment altogether. Further, I have found that many Native clients have not had the opportunity to simply talk to another human being and give form to what they have been through. This may be due to their own reluctance to share their life with others due to mistrust of relationships within their village. As such, I must recognize that if Native clients want to talk, I must let them talk. I do not deter this talking need with techniques that can potentially be a distraction for clients who simply need someone to listen to them for once in their life and, perhaps, for the first time in their life.

Reinforcing the Positive Work of Clients in Context of Historical Trauma

In my clinical practice, clients suffering from full-blown post-traumatic stress disorder or having features of PTSD often describe having preoccupied parents who were emotionally unavailable. This may stem from such parents having their own unresolved traumas on top of struggling with issues of addiction to alcohol and/or other drugs. In any case, my clients are given an understanding of how their own unresolved issues impact a sense of safety and predictability in their own children. Parents suffering from an unhealthy sense of identity, and lacking self-soothing methods for affect regulation, have difficulty maintaining a balanced, grounded perspective when life stressors arise. High levels of anxiety and depression, compounded with feelings of helplessness, consequently can impact their child's developmental progress.

One Native woman, after practicing self-regulation techniques, was able to move through a timeline delineating the micro-events of a particular traumatic memory that had troubled her for several years. Further, she was able to provide a written narrative of that timeline and commented with a smile while writing: "This is the first time I've been able to pay attention to this memory [without avoiding it]." Additionally, the therapeutic work this woman performed was encapsulated within the historical context of trauma to her culture. (She shared how her own parents never took ownership of their alcoholism and the trauma it had masked in their own lives from being raised in boarding schools.) She shared how her drive to become sober and to cope with her past trauma had given her confidence in her ability to be a mother in the future. Up until the time she became sober from alcohol and began working on resolving past trauma, she had no hope for becoming a mother because, she said, "I wouldn't want a child of mine to go through what I had gone through." Now, in a healthy relationship, being sober, and no longer traumatized by her past, she had hope for the future—not only for herself but for her culture and people.

Hence, the individual work my Native clients engage in is not limited to their own life but to the future lives of their children and their children to come. Having this broader picture raises the bar of consciousness and highlights the importance of practicing prosocial behaviors and making the work of Native clients more culturally significant. It is consistent with Freire's (1970) position of empowering oppressed people with a critical consciousness to provide a catalyst for enlightened action. Further, Duran and Duran (1995) assert that the work of therapists will be more effective if the historical issues and their impact on the Native family are validated and acknowledged: "Therapies involving communications, structural, and other systematic approaches can be seen as quite effective if the therapist has knowledge and also validates some of the historical issues that have had a profound intergenerational effect on the Native American family" (158). Transforming traumatic legacies passed down in families over generations has been recognized as an area that traditional therapy, psychiatry, and other interventions have not adequately addressed (Wolynn, 2016).

Case Examples of the 4Rs with Alaska Natives

The following case examples are presented to illustrate the fluid model of the 4Rs. As a mental health provider, I am not rigidly fastened to the four elements. They do, however, create a theoretical template in my mind as I work with Native people. I move with the wind and the waves, in and out of the four elements, depending on the current that my client wants to follow. Sometimes, too, I might not follow one of the elements due to a variety of dynamics that did not guide me toward such a path.

Case #1

Bob, a twenty-seven-year-old Alaska Native man, came voluntarily to me with complaints of fatigue and tendencies toward excessive worrying and thoughts of hurting himself. He explained that he had put off coming to see me for several months because he feared being labeled "crazy" or, worse, fit for placement at a psychiatric facility. I clarified to him, as I often explain to my clients, that my job was not to make his life miserable but rather to support him. Bob had a six-year-old daughter and a supportive relationship with his child's mother. He said that his emotional symptoms had persisted for over five years, and he was tired of getting up each morning fearful of the new day ahead and barely able to get out of bed. In spite of his struggle with lethargy, he was gainfully employed and held a full-time position in his community. He was very interested in learning whether he was depressed or anxious and eagerly accepted the idea of having his emotional and behavioral functioning formally assessed. I had Bob complete the Beck Depression Inventory and the Achenbach Adult Self-Report. Relative to men his age, Bob scored in the clinically significant range for both depression and anxiety as well as somatic problems (e.g., stomachaches, headaches, skin problems); his regular use of alcohol and smoking cannabis placed his substance use in the clinical range as well. (For those clinicians who do not use the aforementioned tools, reading the criteria of the *Diagnostic and Statistical Manual of Mental Disorders [DSM]* for these disorders offers another viable assessment avenue.)

Bob was noticeably relieved when he learned about his levels of depression and anxiety and his tendencies toward somatization. (I have often observed this sense of relief with my Native clients when their emotions are quantified and given a name. The mistrust and stigma of the mental health profession in general can have people misperceiving such services; further, their own alienation from emotions can exaggerate their condition, sometimes making it seem worse than it actually is.) In this case, Bob was relieved to understand that he was not "crazy" after all, that he would not be considered for internment in a mental asylum, and that his depression and anxiety were normal feelings of the human condition that could be worked on. Having his feelings and his sense of overwhelming affect acknowledged and validated brought Bob a sense of relief and also personal empowerment that had been lacking in his life. Most importantly, his enhanced personal agency over his problems led to a high level of motivation toward helping himself.

In the following months, I worked with Bob within the context of individual psychotherapy. As we established rapport and trust, he disclosed significant abuse from his childhood, which he believed contributed substantially to his depression, anxiety, and tendencies toward self-medication via alcohol and using cannabis. In reviewing the cycle of trauma addiction, he could relate to how having intrusive thoughts, feelings, and sensations from previous traumatic experiences rendered a strong desire to find relief or escape from such chronic tension and pain. His method of coping through cannabis and alcohol offered such relief, albeit temporary.

With this understanding, Bob fully endorsed the plan to develop his own battery of self-soothing, grounding strategies for self-rescue from intrusive arousal symptoms that activated his sympathetic nervous system and made his life miserable. He learned diaphragmatic breathing combined with visual imagery of a safe, peaceful place and learned to practice this in session. He also learned to distinguish between "outside danger" and "inside danger" and how to scan his environment when he was feeling anxious or scared to assess if such feelings came from real dangers or internally derived feelings of danger that underscored the need for self-rescue strategies. Bob later added EFT to his personal self-soothing battery and also used it to reinforce and affirm himself.

About one month into individual psychotherapy, Bob chose to reprocess a specific trauma from his childhood that had bothered him ever since it occurred. He provided the metaphor of a movie playing repeatedly throughout his day—consisting of intrusive thoughts, images, and feelings from his past traumatic experiences in childhood—and he wanted desperately for it to go away. Using Gentry's (2014) 5-Narrative Model of Narrative Exposure Therapy (NET), Bob documented the micro-events of the trauma; he also made a written timeline of the event, a pictorial and verbal narrative of the event, followed by a recursive narrative, all the while practicing his self-soothing strategies as his sympathetic nervous system became aroused. Through this procedure, Bob further established a new cognitive interpretation of the trauma—replacing a previous irrational one that had made him feel guilty.

The 5-Narrative Model of NET was completed in one session, about one month into treatment, and it specifically focused on the trauma Bob wanted to address. Interestingly, Bob chose not to engage in NET anymore since he found it to be too emotionally draining and painful. Additionally, he relayed that his level of discomfort from this traumatic event was still a 10 on a scale of 0 to 10.

In spite of this, in subsequent sessions Bob began reporting that his levels of depression were lifting, he was more energetic, and he had a more positive outlook toward his future. Although the "movie" from his traumatic past still played, he was beginning to see his own personal strengths and affirming himself as a valid human being with positive attributes. Additionally, Bob reported less desire to drink alcohol and smoke cannabis. As his individual psychotherapy approached two months, however, he began reporting additional images of past traumas that were emanating from the "movie" playing repeatedly. He became frustrated and elected to try a psychotropic medication to help with his depression and anxiety, but, due to side effects, he quickly gave up the pursuit of medication. During this time, he suffered from what I refer to as an "emotional relapse," where he simply became overwhelmed with feelings, thoughts, and images from his past traumas, and he returned to past coping methods grounded in using substances. This setback was temporary, and Bob recovered quickly—returning to practicing his battery of sober self-soothing strategies. He even adopted another strategy encompassing daily journaling of his thoughts and feelings.

At the nearly three-month mark of receiving weekly individual psychotherapy, Bob began reporting improved mood, less sadness, less lethargy, less anxiety, increased energy, and a positive attitude upon waking up in the morning. Further, all these improved symptoms were accompanied by decreased cravings for alcohol and cannabis. Additionally, he reported becoming more assertive in his life. For example, he was able to let his colleagues know his needs, and this assertiveness extended to family members as well. Moreover, he was reengaged in activities such as fishing and hunting that had previously brought him pleasure. After the three-month mark, Bob's "movie" of past traumas that had intruded daily was no longer

offering an interpretation, I continued to listen as Fay shared further awareness about herself. Specifically, she was astounded by the realization that she had been medicating her feelings and thoughts of her past through her use of alcohol. She could clearly link that alcohol blocked out her remembering the trauma of her childhood. Now, in her efforts to become sober, her childhood memories were returning.

Fay became angry. "That fucking God-damned pedophile!" she yelled as she stood up and paced my office. "I'm going to kill him!" Since I knew the individual she was referring to was still living in the village, I was acutely aware that Fay's desire to "kill" was a real possibility, particularly given the enormous amount of anger she was demonstrating—anger I had never witnessed before and that quite shocked me, given Fay's usual calm and passive demeanor. I sat on the edge of my chair and asked Fay to calm down. I led her in diaphragmatic breathing, telling her that this was a time to use her calming strategies. I told her that she had every right to be angry, that her feelings were justified and valid, but that she needed to use her angry energy to guide herself in a positive direction. I spoke to her candidly about what would happen if she were to act on her anger and kill her perpetrator—it would only serve to disempower her, since she would likely go to jail. I asserted, though, that Fay had other choices to channel her anger. She sat down, and we talked about her options: going to the village police, to the state troopers, and filing a report. And then Fay began sobbing uncontrollably. During this time, she shared her dismay of how she had "ruined" her life by drinking alcohol and smoking pot. "I've done nothing," she stated, mired in feelings of helplessness. She shared how the introduction of alcohol to her culture disempowered it just like it had disempowered her. I shared with Fay that for the first time I was observing "the real Fay," the Fay with real feelings, and that—in spite of the pain she was experiencing—I was honored to witness the work she was doing. Further, I shared with her that if she made a report to the authorities, I would be there to support her. Additionally,

I reinforced to her that she was still young, that she still had a life to live, she still had the opportunity to reclaim her personal power just like her own culture was reclaiming power in many ways.

Fay laughed, telling me, to my surprise, that she had already made a report to the authorities earlier in the day. I thanked her for telling me this and told her I would follow up with the authorities myself. Fay supported this plan. Moreover, she shared with me that she did not intend to actually kill her perpetrator. Although she certainly felt like killing him, she realized she had to take more charge of her life and start doing something with it instead of drinking and smoking. Within two weeks, an investigation was under way with the reports Fay and I had made with the authorities. Further, Fay became energized into action. She decided to move to a town with a sober relative on the road system. Two weeks after that, I received information from Fay that she was working full-time and was attending outpatient substance abuse treatment that catered to clients with comorbid issues such as substance abuse and past trauma.

Although I never engaged Fay in exposure therapy, she nonetheless reprocessed trauma in the context of a caring therapeutic alliance. Her case is a nice example of how a positive therapeutic relationship can enter into a client's development when such development has been derailed. Fay's development, during her period of alcohol use, had plateaued into a state of feeling ineffectual, powerless, helpless. The therapeutic relationship, enamored with motivational interviewing elements supporting Fay's sobriety combined with teaching some self-regulatory techniques, provided emotional attunement that allowed Fay to express past trauma and transmute it into a more useful form (i.e., making a report to authorities, energizing her, using her angry energy to assume positive control of her life). This was all made more meaningful, and more poignant, under the rubric of acculturation and the disempowering dynamic of alcohol on Fay's people and her own life.

Initial Treatment Engagement

It is not uncommon for clients to meet me once or twice and not be seen for a month or more. A young Native man came to me in crisis, and we addressed his issues in two sessions, and then I did not see him again for over two months. I wondered if I had done anything to discourage him from continuing treatment. So I was surprised to receive a phone call from him two months later, requesting an appointment to see me again. When we met, I asked him if I had done anything to discourage him from seeing me, since we had not met for so long. He was taken aback. Rather, he explained that he had been busy; attending sessions was not a priority, particularly since he was no longer in crisis. He also shared that he was getting what he wanted from treatment; having sessions every one or two months was meeting his needs.

It is important to recognize that with some clients, particularly those whose cultural beliefs can impact treatment, therapy consisting of dozens of sessions over a six-month period or more is not likely. Rather, it is common for a multicultural client to come in for one or two therapy sessions (Sue and Zane 1987). This is not necessarily a sign of treatment failure.

My initial sessions with Alaska Natives are consistent with Comas-Diaz's (2012) concept of considering clients as consultants. When I first meet with a client, I do not bury them in Medicaid paperwork but rather focus on meeting their needs and resonating with what brought them in to see me. Through empathy, active listening, affective attunement, cultural resonance, and collaboration, I form a therapeutic alliance that often leads clients to desire continued services. Clients often tell me that the respect and genuine caring I show them is very healing and a motivating dynamic to stay in treatment. Also, normalizing their mental health problems reduces the stigma of treatment.

Parenting and the Use of Parent-Child Interaction Therapy (PCIT)

One of the results of the ACEs study underscored the importance for individuals—particularly those who score high on the ACEs questionnaire—to learn positive parenting techniques. The thesis is: if an individual has experienced horrendous parenting as a child, then that individual, if they become a parent, probably would benefit from some positive parenting education. Parent-child interaction therapy (PCIT) is one method that can be taught to parents to promote better listening skills and attunement to their two-to-seven-year-old children (Hembree-Kigin and McNeil 1995). It has been used successfully by Native Americans and Alaska Natives (Bigfoot and Funderburk 2011). I have found it to be an effective method for use with parents interested in learning additional tools to add to their parenting repertoire. I have also taught this technique to several Head Start programs and their staff, including the parents they work with.

When I first began using PCIT over twenty years ago, I thought I needed all the high-tech equipment: I invested in a one-way mirror and a "bug-in-the-ear" system for communicating to parents as they play with their child. Since then, I have found that this method can be taught in a small office space with simply the therapist providing verbal feedback to parents when they begin trying this technique that teaches them to see the world through children's eyes, moving at their pace while paying keen attention to their behavior and thoughts and reinforcing the positive things they do. I have found that children are not disturbed by my making comments to their parents while they play. PCIT has been found to be an effective method for enhancing parenting skills and reducing problematic behavior in children (Schuhmann et al. 2010) and has been successfully used cross-culturally (see, for example, Leung et al. 2015).

I recall working with a four-year-old boy who was quite defiant and oppositional toward his parents, particularly his mother. Having the luxury of a large playroom at the time, I worked with the boy within the context of doing PCIT in the playroom while his mother quietly watched. After I had worked with the boy for about twenty minutes, I had him play by himself while I talked with his mother in my office. I reviewed with the mother what she had witnessed. I used this opportunity, like I habitually do when teaching parents this technique, to review the elements of PCIT: *Describing* verbally to the child his prosocial behavior ("I see you now grabbing the truck and making it pull the cars"); *reflecting* any verbalizations the child makes ("Yes, that truck has to move slowly pulling all those cars"); *imitating* appropriate play ("Well, I think I'm going to join you and try out this blue truck for myself"); and *praising* specific prosocial behaviors the child demonstrates ("I like how you carefully pull those cars"). In the next session, when the mother was ready, I had her engage her son in PCIT in the playroom while I watched. When the mother got stuck, I gave her some suggestions but without taking over.

After several weeks of PCIT, this mother became proficient in this method with her boy. More importantly, her son's initially defiant and oppositional behavior declined significantly. Because her husband worked long hours, unfortunately he could not attend these sessions. However, I gave the mother "homework" to have her husband observe her doing the technique with their son at least five minutes per day.

I am consistently amazed how giving children a little bit of special attention every day helps them feel validated and worthwhile, and helps promote their positive emotional and behavioral growth. The four-year-old boy in this case, for example, was so excited to come to his play sessions with his mother. In one session, the mother commented to me that during the previous week she had thought her son was regressing when he became quite angry because he had lost his "timer." She did not know what he meant by "timer" until it dawned on her that he was referring to his appointment card I regularly gave him upon leaving my office. Once his appointment card was found, he became calm and cooperative.

Too often (and I admit, as a parent, I am guilty of this as well) parents pay attention only to their children's bad behavior without reinforcing the positive choices their children are making. Parent-child interaction therapy offers a medium of positive interaction that can quickly usurp the negativity between a parent and a child. It also is a fun technique that allows adults to see the world through their child's eyes and appreciate their unique attributes.

I once worked with a mother and son who did not make a good fit: the mother was used to hurrying and getting things done, while her son was slow and methodical when approaching the world. Through PCIT, the mother learned that she had to slow down, becoming mindful of her own tendencies to rush through life, when relating to her boy. Furthermore, she came to appreciate her son's unique traits: he was inquisitive and thoughtful, carefully exploring the playroom and its contents before selecting a toy to engage in. And even when he selected a toy, he was again very methodical in his implementation of the toy. The mother, through PCIT, came to be less impatient with her boy and more adept at recognizing, appreciating, and commenting on her son's strengths. She also became more sensitive to her own issues of needing to control the pace of things happening around her, especially in the context of parenting. She learned to slow down—becoming more attuned to the process of "being" rather than "doing."

Strengths Perspective

Malcolm Forbes, the billionaire publisher, coined the phrase "He who dies with the most toys, wins." His lavish lifestyle, filled with parties, travel, and a collection of homes, yachts, aircraft, art, motorcycles, and Fabergé eggs, reflected what many people in the Western world want: prosperity, power, and privilege. Consumerism, though, and its concomitant problems of debt, depression, anxiety, obesity, addictions, and unhappiness, has been well-documented in the literature (Chatzky 2003; de Graaf, Waan, and Naylor 2005; Hamilton and Denniss 2005). Conversely, the strengths and values that often have been highlighted among Indigenous peoples are their generosity and mutual bond toward helping one another. Waller's (2006) observations of Indigenous peoples include: "A family's wealth and status are measured not in terms of what family members possess, but by their generosity to others" (52).

Once, while blizzard-bound over the New Year's holiday in the Iñupiat community of Elim, I was welcomed at their annual New Year's Eve feast, where community residents met to socialize and eat a fabulous meal. While dining on reindeer stew, reindeer ribs, and *akutaq* (Eskimo ice cream, a well-known Alaska Native favorite made for special occasions and typically made with Crisco, berries, ground fish, or seal oil), I felt honored to be among these Alaska Natives whose generosity and goodwill I much appreciated during the separation from my own family on this holiday. As I dined, I felt the spirit of generosity I have observed throughout years of living and working among Alaska Natives in the Bering Strait region and Norton Sound. As I mentioned earlier, I have consistently observed that—in spite of family feuds that may exist within a Native community—when a tragedy strikes, people pull together and differences seem to melt away in lieu of individuals and families supporting those who are experiencing hardship. I knew that the generosity I experienced during that New Year's Eve community feast existed over a century ago in Alaska Native communities in the Bering Strait region. I recalled how, in the 1800s for example, Alaska Natives enacted their goodwill to the crews of whaling ships helplessly stuck in the ice and saved the crews' lives in the stark arctic winter through their generosity.

The strengths of Alaska Natives and other Indigenous peoples have not gone away. Further, the mental health and social work professions cater to the strengths perspective, yet mental health and social science are historically infused with a medical mindset that highlights the pathology of people and minimizes their inherent capacities to function successfully (Schon 1987). Given such a bias,

Waller (2006) asserts: "With professional helpers whose model is a conglomeration of negative stereotypes, who needs enemies?" (47).

Marginalized people are prone to being labeled deviant or lacking self-determination and autonomy due to their decreased social power (Saleebey 1997). As mental health providers, we can counter this unproductive bias by arming ourselves with a vocabulary that celebrates and accents the inherent attributes and strengths in all human beings. If we truly endorse the principle of self-determination, we must talk and walk in the spirit of self-determination with the Native people we work with. A strengths-based approach that is respectful and empowering is consistent with our work with Alaska Natives. Table 1 contrasts the strengths model with traditional medical/rehabilitative models of helping (Saleebey 1997, 119), where patients are considered passive recipients of provider-directed care.

It is incumbent upon mental health providers to be mindful of the strengths perspective with all of our clients but particularly with disenfranchised individuals such as Indigenous peoples who historically have been disempowered. Adhering to a medical model mindset heightens our potential to promote dependency rather self-determination. Being mindful of the differences between the strengths perspective and the medical model described in Table 1, we can monitor our own behavior to help gauge whether our work is bent toward promoting dependency or self-determination. Further, following a medical mindset potentially serves as a colonizing pattern of behavior.

Kaplan and Girard (1994) maintain:

> People are more motivated to change when their strengths are supported. Instead of asking family members what their problems are, a worker can ask what strengths they bring to the family and what they think are the strengths of other family members. Through this process the worker helps the family discover its capabilities and formulate a new way to think about

Table 1. The Strengths model contrasted with traditional medical/ rehabilitative models of helping.

Factor	Strengths Model	Medical/ Rehabilitative Models
Value base	Human potential to grow, heal, learn Human ability to identify wants Self-determination Strengths of person and environment Individuality and uniqueness	Problem resolution dependent upon professional expertise Compliance with prescribed treatments Patient lacks insight and knowledge about health
Focus	Combining personal and environmental resources to create situations for personal goal achievement	Professional diagnosis to determine the specific nature of the person's problem and to prescribe treatment
Solution to problems	Determined by consumer/ environment Natural community resources used first Consumer authority and investment	Professional-oriented assessment and service delivery
Social and cultural role	Consumer "Elders taking care of themselves"	Patient "Taking care of the elderly"
Case management relationship	Consumer choice and decision making Develops rapport and trust Case manager coaches, supports, and encourages Case manager replaces self when possible with natural helpers	Clients are passive recipients Professional contact limited to assessment, planning, evaluating functions Provider-directed decision making and interventions
Case management tasks	Identifying strengths and resources Rejuvenating and creating natural helping networks Developing relationships Provided within daily routines	Teaching skills to overcome deficits Monitoring compliance Medical management of identified problems
Desired client outcomes	Interdependence Quality of life Self-efficacy Consumer satisfaction	Problem resolution Maximum bodily functioning Meeting identified biomedical standards of treatment

Dennis Saleebey, *The Strengths Perspective in Social Work Practice, 2nd Ed.*, (New York: Pearson, 1997). Reprinted by permission of Pearson Education, Inc.

themselves. . . . The worker creates a language of strength, hope and movement. (53)

Saleebey (2006) delineates some of the elements of the strengths perspective in practice:

- As clients initially share their pain, stress, loss/trauma, mental health providers need to listen for hints of resiliency, inner capacity, will, for coping and rebounding;
- The mental health practitioner stimulates a narrative of resiliency and strength by providing "the words and images of strengths, wholeness, and capacity;"
- The capacities and resilient aspects of the client are linked to the individual's hopes, goals and visions and to relevant resources in their environment;
- Through a collaborative process, the mental health provider and client consolidate the strengths that have been accented and a new capacity to activate resources within the client and within his/her environment. (88–90)

Duncan, Hubble, and Miller (1997) eloquently describe the strengths perspective in this manner:

We have learned to listen more, turn off the intervention spigot, stay still, direct our attention to them [the client]—recalling, as Ram Dass once said: "The quieter you become the more you will hear." The greater success we have experienced in doing this, the more room clients have had to be themselves, use their own resources, discover possibilities, attribute self-enhancing meanings to their actions, and take responsibility. (207)

Solution-focused therapy is a viable method for operationalizing the strengths model. It involves a process whereby Native people determine for themselves where they want to go and how they want to go. It uses a vocabulary that affirms their abilities and capacities to choose and deal with the consequences of their choices. Moreover, it is an active approach that involves the individual in solving their own problems. Numerous materials detail this approach (Berg 1994; Berg and Reuss 1998; Berg and de Shazer 1994; DeJong and Berg 1998; Kraal and Kowalski 1989; Saleebey 1997, 2006).

Berg and de Shazer (1994) identify specific questions that serve as "taps on the shoulder" for the client to move forward and find solutions to problems they wish to focus on. Within this format, they perceive clients as designing their own treatment plan with their own treatment goals in lieu of traditional therapy, which focuses on the therapist as the expert who makes a diagnosis about what is wrong with the client and identifies what is needed to make their life better. Some central questions they have formulated are:

1. Pre-treatment change questions. Frequently, clients report a positive change between the time they call us for an appointment and our first meeting. It is important to explore with clients in the first meeting if this was true for them. It not only helps identify what issues they may be working on but also accents the positive things they already are doing to feel and be successful.

2. The miracle question. This question is asked as follows: "Suppose when you go to sleep tonight, a miracle happens and the problems that brought you here today are solved. But since you are asleep, you can't know this miracle has happened until you wake up tomorrow. What will be different tomorrow that will let you know this miracle has happened and the problem is solved?" This question helps transition clients to looking at solutions to the specific problems that brought them in for treatment. It is important for the therapist to allow ample moments of silence so the client can think. And it is important to not accept answers of "I don't know."

3. Exception questions. These questions follow the miracle question, such as saying: "When did little pieces of this miracle happen for you?" When the client acknowledges times when the "miracle" happened, possible follow-up questions might be: "How did that happen? What did you do to make that happen? What do you need to do to make that happen routinely for you?"

4. Scaling questions. A scale of 1 to 10 or 0 to 10 is used to quantify the client's own assessment of their motivation, hopefulness, progress, confidence, and a host of other factors that are related to solutions to the identified problem. For example, if a client identifies that they are a "2" with regard to maintaining sobriety, follow-up questions might be: "When was your score higher? What were you doing at that time to make your score higher? What do you need to do now to raise your current score?" I have found scaling questions very useful to gauge how a client's week went and what a client might do to maintain their score or raise it. Further, scaling questions are very useful for clients who are not verbal: drawing a scale from 0 to 10, for example, can allow clients to pick where they are, and this can be a starting point for a session.

5. The nightmare question. Berg and Reuss (1998) added this question in their work with substance abuse clients. They believe it is safer to help a client imagine "hitting bottom" than to actually hit bottom. The question is presented as follows: "Suppose that when you go to bed tonight, sometime in the middle of the night a nightmare occurs. In this nightmare all the problems that brought you here suddenly get as bad as they can possibly get. This would be a nightmare. But this nightmare comes true. What would you notice tomorrow morning that would let you know you were living a nightmare life?" Follow-up questions might include: "Are there times now when small pieces of this nightmare are happening? What is the nightmare like during these times? What would it take to prevent this nightmare from happening? How

confident are you that you can do what it takes to keep it from happening? What things have you done to keep this nightmare from happening so far?"

6. Coping questions. These questions are often used with dying clients or clients who have difficulty making progress and for whom treatment does not seem to make a difference. Coping questions might include: "How have you managed to cope this far? What are the things you do to help yourself manage? How do you do that? What do you have to do to keep doing that? How come it is not worse? How are you doing as well as you are?"

The aforementioned solution-focused questions can be superimposed on Saleebey's (2006) schema of strengths-based practice summarized in Figure 2. Working with a client's internal and external resources, fueled by their hopes and dreams and goals, therapists can support their clients on a strengths-driven path where clients make decisions, encapsulating their strengths and resources, as the therapeutic process collaboratively moves toward a better future.

Motivational interviewing (Miller and Rollnick 2002) is also consistent with the strengths perspective. I have found it particularly useful for working with people who initially are not willing to address substance use problems. It is a collaborative rather than confrontational approach, and it is compatible with respecting the dignity and worth of the individual. Recent efforts have made it culturally applicable to Alaska Natives (see Tomlin et al. 2014); this user-friendly manual is not only applicable for working with Native clients with substance abuse problems but underscores strategies to help individuals struggling with problematic behaviors toward self-motivation and positive change. Some fundamental methods for effecting healthy change include expressing empathy, developing discrepancy, rolling with a client's resistance, and supporting self efficacy (Tomlin et al. 2014, 21–22).

Trauma-Focused Narrative Therapy with Children

Although the aforementioned narrative exposure therapy method can be used with children, I have found that engaging children in making a story of their experience with trauma is helpful. A five-year-old girl was brought to me by her parents from her village to the hub community of Nome, where I had been working. She was engaged in creating a story of her life that included her experience of losing a friend who was carried away by the river current she was playing in.

This child enjoyed drawing, so she was highly motivated to make a pictorial narrative of her life. In this method, she was initially engaged in drawing pictures of where she lived in her village, her friends there, and her habitual activities. I helped her put words to the pictures as well ("This is my friend X. We are playing . . . "). The images of her life in the village gradually led to her experience of playing with her friend in the river. Other pictures followed, depicting her friend being suddenly carried away by the river. She drew herself and how she felt when this happened. She also drew herself when she learned that her friend had drowned and her body was found several days later. Pictures followed of her life without her friend and how she coped with her loss.

This process of creating a pictorial and narrative story can take several sessions to complete. It is a safe, structured way for a child to narrate their trauma through the gradual creation of pictures and words. Once a child's story is complete, they read the story to their parents, and then the parents likewise read the story to the child. In this process, the child provides a verbal narration to their trauma, like NET, but there also is a recursive narrative when the parents read the story as well. Other family members and extended family can be involved in this process to provide the child with even more validation and support. This approach, moreover, appears similar to trauma-focused cognitive-behavioral therapy advocated for use

Figure 2. The elements of strengths-based practice

RISK FACTORS			PROTECTIVE/GENERATIVE FACTORS		
Challenges			***Resources***		
Damage Trauma Disorder Stress	Internal and external	**+**	Strengths Capacities Talents Gifts	Internal and external	→
Expectations/possibilities			***Decisions***		
Hopes Dreams Visions Goals Self-righting		→	Choices and options about paths to be taken Defining opportunities and setting directions Gathering resources and mobilizing strengths		→
Project					
Mutual collaboration in work toward		→	A better future		

Dennis Saleebey, *The Strengths Perspective in Social Work Practice, 4th Ed.* (New York: Pearson, 2006). Reprinted by permission of Pearson Education, Inc.

among Native children (Bigfoot 2011; Bigfoot and Schmidt 2010). Additionally, once a child's story is created, they can take it home and read it with the guided support of their parents. In this manner, having a tangible "book" of a child's life provides the opportunity for repeated and supportive exposure to the child's trauma.

Crisis Intervention

Social psychology has criticized psychological debriefing, such as critical incident stress debriefing (CISD), due to its wide acceptance and implementation "before social scientists conducted rigorous tests of its effectiveness" (Aronson, Wilson, and Akert 2013). At first glance, the method appears intuitively sound: if people who experience a traumatic event are helped to talk about it shortly thereafter, they can render a cathartic experience to prevent later psychiatric symptoms, including post-traumatic stress disorder (PTSD). CISD has often been used with fire and police departments, and many counselors who came to the aid of people following the September 11, 2001, terrorist attacks also employed this technique. After a comprehensive review of the literature, however, Harvard psychologist Richard McNally and his colleagues (2003) concluded that there is "no convincing evidence" that psychological debriefing methods prevent post-traumatic stress disorder (72). In spite of this, CISD continues to receive support for its use among first responders to traumatic events (see, for example, Riddell and Clouse 2004). Mitchell (2003) argues that some reviews of CISD—including that of McNally et. al. (2003)—have generated a number of misconceptions that have blatantly and unfairly characterized the field of crisis intervention. His 2003 article identifies some of the most common misconceptions while offering arguments countering such errors. Too, Mitchell (2004) delineates guidelines for early intervention programs that offer the best potential for providing effective early crisis intervention services.

The current discussion is not intended to set the record straight concerning the controversy with CISD. I have been called to do CISD many times, particularly with medical providers who were first responders to a traumatic event such as suicide. I have no problems accepting invitations to meet with first responders to a human tragedy when called upon to do so in a Native community. But I do have difficulty traveling out to a community when requests to do crisis services are generated from the hub community rather than from the village where the crisis has originated. It is important that requests for crisis intervention are generated from within a community rather than from outside, lest we impose agendas that Native communities do not want. I have found Mitchell's model of CISD (Mitchell 1983, 1988; www.info-trauma.org) most effective and practical, and other crisis responders have had similar reactions (see, for example, Pack 2012).

Often, CISD is referred to behavioral health staff by medical supervisors overseeing staff at the clinics in the villages. As such, it is often presented as an external solution toward supporting first responders to crises in the villages. Because of this external delivery, when conducting CISD sessions I see my role as a mental health professional to internalize and reinforce the inherent strengths of individuals and communities rather than emphasizing dependency on CISD sessions to promote healthy functioning and recovery. Consistent with working with Alaska Natives in the spirit of self-determination, I stress during CISD sessions the uniqueness of each individual's response to crisis and how each individual is the "expert" in their own recovery process. I acknowledge the natural recovery process that occurs with individuals and communities and that tapping into existing strengths and support systems is more important than my coming to do a "debriefing" session that is outside of their natural support system, that is external rather than internal to their support network. Although I do provide psychoeducation on such things as acute stress disorder and make myself available for future counseling sessions should anyone desire to access such services, I take the time to have participants identify the strengths inherent in themselves and their communities that they rely upon during times of crisis. I also acknowledge the importance of colleagues being mindful as they support one another in the aftermath of a human tragedy. For further reading, Slawinski (2005) endorses a strengths-based approach to crisis response that focuses on natural recovery processes.

Moreover, when conducting CISD, I emphasize that no one in the meeting should feel forced to talk, that sometimes people need time to distance themselves from the event they have just experienced, and this is not a pathological defense mechanism indicative of denial or avoidance but rather a healthy way to cope with tragedy. I also emphasize that no one should attempt to shame such individuals or outcast them in any way for their decision to not participate. Working in this manner, this method is more in line with providing psychological first aid (see World Health Organization 2011) and its components advocating practical care and support that does not intrude, listening to people but not pressuring them to talk, and comforting people and helping them feel calm.

Further, consistent with PART (see the section on "Relational-Cultural Therapy and Multicultural Care"), the importance of physical presence during crisis intervention should not be underestimated. Sitting in the waiting room of a village clinic after a crisis response, for example, and showing receptiveness and availability to others is useful. In one village, where I supported a number of first responders to a tragic event, I was encouraged by one professional to simply walk the village to let people know that I was present and available. When visiting a home whose family has lost a loved one, I may simply sit with people without doing any formal intervention. Physical presence from supportive outsiders can have a reassuring, comforting effect on people suffering from loss and/or trauma. And, again, it is consistent with providing psychological first aid.

Psychotropic Medication

I am against extremist views when considering the use of psychotropic medications with Alaska Natives, or any other clients for that matter: I have met mental health and medical providers who advocate that all psychiatric medications should be avoided, and I have met mental health and medical providers who are quick to medicate any symptoms suggesting depression or discomfort. Using discretion when making a psychiatric referral for possible medication is warranted. Such referrals need to be conducted in collaboration with our clients and not imposed on them like a mandate.

It is important, too, that if a mental health provider makes a referral to a medical provider, medical factors should be ruled out before psychotropic medications are considered. Various medical conditions (e.g., anemia, heart disease, thyroid problems) can affect mental health. Additionally, there are numerous nutritional deficiencies (e.g., omega-3 fatty acid deficiency, vitamin D and B deficiency) that may cause depression. When I make a referral to a medical provider for considering a client for psychotropic medication, I routinely ask that a complete blood count be performed first. Additionally, we must not forget other factors that can contribute to depression, such as alcohol and drug abuse and the effects of certain medications our clients may be taking.

We must also be mindful, as Mehl-Madrona (2007) maintains, that "psychiatric drugs do not cure poverty, homelessness, isolation, or loneliness" (24). Still, there are individuals who can and do benefit from psychotropic medications. A depressed client, for example, who demonstrated all the neuro-vegetative symptoms of a biological depression, was doing all the right things in her life: trying to get a good amount of sleep, exercising, and eating right, yet she could not shake the deep depression that she suffered with. She wanted to try a medical option and was referred to our psychiatrist, who prescribed a selective serotonin reuptake inhibitor (SSRI). In the weeks and months that followed—consisting of psychotherapy and medication monitoring—her symptoms improved greatly: she was no longer preoccupied with morbid thoughts of death, had increased energy and mood, was sleeping well, and was balancing her life with exercise and other healthy activities such as starting her own business. Within one year, this woman wanted to be removed from her medication. I supported this decision, and she continues to function effectively to date.

Yet psychiatry can impart an intimidating and colonizing influence. I worked with a Native client who made positive gains in psychotherapy with his symptoms of post-traumatic stress disorder. He moved out of the region and went to live in a part of Alaska that did not have village-based mental health services in his new community. When he experienced stress, exacerbated by being isolated, he accessed telemedicine services via a private mental health facility in Anchorage, and he was immediately instructed by the psychiatrist to be placed on psychotropic medications. This client resisted such instructions. He called me at my office and explained that he believed he was doing relatively well, was practicing some healthy thinking and behavioral strategies to cope with life, but he simply wanted someone to talk to due to the tremendous isolation he was feeling in his current living situation. The psychiatrist he interacted with via telemedicine services was not hearing him, he told me; and he felt obligated to go on psychotropic medications because it was being presented as a medical mandate. I told him that he was in charge of what medicines entered his body, not some doctor practicing in Anchorage. I encouraged him to again reiterate to his psychiatrist what he needed, that he was not looking for medication. Two weeks later, he called to let me know that he was now talking with a mental health clinician and that his psychiatrist had finally listened to what services he was requesting.

Being sensitive to alternative methods for helping clients feel better and function better promotes their autonomy in the process of healing. Some parents, for example, are adamantly against medicating their children's ADD/ADHD. I strive to educate parents about their choices for treatment: possible medications versus nonmedication approaches (see, for example, Burdick 2016); I also stress that, if medications are tried, this is simply a trial run to see if it is helpful. That is, their child is not sentenced to a life on medications. Some depressed clients may pursue nutritional supplements as a method to mitigate their depression in lieu of psychotropic medications. This needs to be respected. An excellent resource for clients interested in nutritional treatments to improve mental health disorders comes from the naturopathic physician Anne Procyk (2018). Leslie Korn, a Harvard Medical School–trained traumatologist specializing in mental health nutrition and integrative approaches to treating the mind and the body, offers another resource in her book *Eat Right, Feel Right: Over 80 Recipes and Tips to Improve Mood, Sleep, Attention and Focus* (2017).

Bibliotherapy

We must not forget using bibliotherapy, or book therapy, as an adjunctive service to our mental health practices in a Native community. Giving our Native clients a copy, for example, of Harold Napoleon's *Yuuyaraq: The Way of the Human Being* (1996) can help reinforce consciousness-raising regarding historical trauma. Other books that have been helpful: for clients dealing with sexual abuse, *Invisible Girls* (Feuereisen 2005); for rape victims, *Resurrection After Rape* (Atkinson 2010); and for adult children of alcoholics, *Adult Children of Alcoholics* (Woititz 1983).

Bibliotherapy can encourage a therapeutic response for those clients who enjoy reading. Moreover, it can help individuals of all ages—children, adults, and seniors—deal with a wide range of physical, emotional, and social issues. Sometimes, too, it can simply help with forming a culturally sensitive therapeutic alliance. I recall working with an Elder who loved to read historical fiction on Alaska Natives; she appreciated my giving her a copy of *Ashana* (Roesch 1990), one of my favorites, and this helped our engagement in a productive therapeutic alliance.

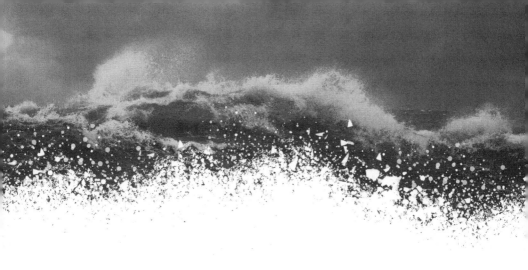

Adjunctive Considerations

The following considerations of the author's model are no less important than the ones discussed in previous chapters. Rather, the concepts delineated complement the preceding discussions and can be used to augment therapeutic work with Alaska Natives. Some topics covered here are not discussed in depth (e.g., Stages of Changes, Community Readiness Model); it is assumed the reader already has some familiarity with them. However, references are provided for the reader to pursue additional information.

Self-Determination Versus Dependency

We are cognizant of the Native drive toward self-determination and empowerment, due to historical forces that have disempowered them in a multitude of ways. We exercise compassion for behaviors that are consistent with helping Alaska Natives achieve self-determination, particularly in the context of their mental health and overall sense of wellness. While we may be passionate about what we do as mental health professionals, such energy is tempered by our compassion. Whitfield (2010), who eloquently describes healthy relationships versus unhealthy relationships, states in his book *Boundaries and Relationships*:

> in true compassion we feel warm and caring and yet do not feel compelled to jump in and rescue, fix or try to heal them. We are still there for people if they reach out to us in any way; but we are secure enough in ourself not to try to use fixing them to fill our own emptiness. (108)

He goes on to explain: "If we are attached to the outcome and try to fix or rescue the other person, we are not practicing compassion. We are in a more primitive state of consciousness that we can call *passion*" (109). Further, a person who does not exercise healthy boundaries and seeks to fix, rescue, change, or control another individual is engaged in codependence.

Figure 3 offers a visual medium for understanding the dance we do as mental health providers in a Native community. Having healthy boundaries is essential. We can simply review the legacy of outsiders who have come into "Native Country" with the intent of doing "good things," only to have such "good things" lead to Native people becoming dependent, disenfranchised, disempowered, and traumatized with an acute loss of personal ego strength, dignity, and agency. Figure 3 reminds us of the walk we are doing while in a Native community: exercising behaviors and conduct that are filled with passion but tempered with the caring boundaries of compassion. We can still be passionate about what we do, but we must hold true to the caring and grounded boundaries of compassion where we are not in a hurry to "fix things."

This walk is similar to my canoe experience on the Bering Sea. As I became more passionate about reaching Stuart Island and/or the mainland of Stebbins, I engaged in frantic behavior involving paddling as hard as I could without any thought of what I was doing save for my goal of reaching land. This behavior made things worse—almost leading me to capsize. Yet, as I calmed down and became more mindful of the ocean and the wind, I was able to conduct myself in a more meaningful manner that allowed me to reach land. I exercised compassion with my canoe while respecting the boundaries it offered as well as the boundaries offered by the wind and the waves. And I achieved self determination, positive progress toward land, without becoming enmeshed with the wind and the waves. Without such care and attention to these dynamics, I was a lost soul, and my experience on the Bering Sea would certainly have ended tragically.

Dependency Patterns

I was once approached by a Native woman in her village who asked me if she could conduct a healing circle within her own community. I was taken aback by this encounter. Here I was, an outsider to this woman's home community, yet I was being asked permission to conduct a traditional activity to help her own people.

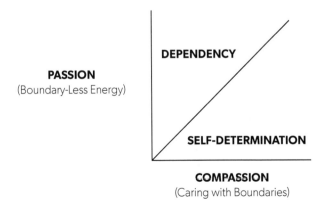

Figure 3. Self-Determination versus Dependency

I speak of the above experience not to be condescending toward the Native woman who approached me. Rather, I discuss it because I believe it is an example of one type of dependency pattern—psychological dependency—that has gradually evolved over one hundred years with some Native people. It is another example of Native disempowerment in the form of an external locus of control. Most importantly, it underscores how non-Native mental health providers must be aware of such dependency patterns and not participate in reinforcing and promoting them.

I could have been proud that this Native woman viewed me as a powerful person who was a vital resource in initiating activities to help her people. I could have basked in the affirmation—validating my professional skills and status. I could have called my colleagues and told them about it, that it was a clear indication that I was doing a good job out here in the village. I could have reinforced the woman's external way of looking at things and tell her that by all means I give her permission to do such activities.

Instead, however, I talked with her about how she did not have to ask me for permission to do talking circles in her community, that she had every right to begin these by herself, that she had every right to help her own people without my approval, although I certainly would offer my support should she desire it. I emphasized that the community she was living in was her own, and that I was an outsider, a guest. I stressed that she had every right to do talking circles with her people and that no outsider had the right to discourage such efforts. Further, I shared with her that I saw other Native people in other villages doing talking circles that the community perceived as very positive and helpful, and that I would be happy to put her in contact with them so they could offer their own expertise.

In another Native community, a traditional village dance—involving their own drummers and dancers—was nearly called off when a motivational speaker from Anchorage canceled his trip. When community leaders decided to push ahead and have the scheduled dance, they asked me to say something prior to the dance. I shared how, yes, we were all disappointed that the speaker from Anchorage had unfortunately canceled. But I also emphasized that I knew this Native community was capable of doing their own motivational community meetings. Further, the Anchorage speaker's absence provided an opportunity for the community to show its strength by doing motivational activities themselves.

The traditional village dance proceeded and was highly successful, charged with an electrical energy that carried a positive spirit of hope and well-being. Some outsiders attending this event to observe the Native community's traditional dance were in tears when asked to share their perceptions of it. During the ceremony, one community leader reiterated what I had said: "We can do this ourselves without relying on others."

Again, as outside mental health providers, we must be cognizant of dependency thinking and behaviors in the Native people among whom we live and work. With such awareness, we can correct misconceptions that Native people must be dependent on outside sources of support. We can reinforce and promote the spirit of self-determination in patterns of Native thinking and behavior.

Colonization Patterns

Colonization has been defined as "the process of forcing one's own culture on another by means of subjugation and exploitation" (Butler et al. 2005). The collective trauma encompassing colonization effects on Alaska Natives must be at the forefront of awareness for mental health providers working with Alaska Native communities. Further, we must be sensitive to existing colonizing patterns so that we do not participate in and perpetuate their execution. Some colonization patterns I have observed in Alaska Native communities are discussed here.

Lack of Awareness of and Respect for Native Resources

Outsiders not respecting or being mindful of the village-based resources a Native community offers is one example of a colonizing
pattern. I was once called out on a crisis to a Native village where
a child had lost both parents and was being cared for by grandparents. A worker from the Office of Children's Services (OCS) flew
out to the village the next day, and a meeting was convened with me
and the village police officer. The OCS worker shared the plan to
remove the child from the village due to the view that the child was
not being adequately cared for by their relatives. The OCS worker
stated that the child being allowed to attend school the day after
their parents died was a clear act of negligence, because the child
was not being allowed to grieve properly. The village police officer
and I shared our concerns that removing the child from their home
community was not in the child's best interests and would probably
exacerbate the grieving process because the child would be forced
to live with a strange foster family in a strange land (Anchorage).
Further, the village police officer maintained that the child attending school on the day after losing their parents was probably the best
thing, since the school had always been a safe, secure, and structured haven for the child. I asked if the OCS worker had consult-
ed with the village ICWA worker. The caseworker stated that they
had not. Since the ICWA worker was out of town, she was promptly
reached on her cell phone. Once she learned about the OCS plan to
remove the child from the village, she became irate and stated that
under no circumstances would she agree with such a plan, that the
child would remain in her village under the care and custody of the
grandparents.

Language

I often hear itinerant mental health providers who travel to a Native
village refer to the village they work in as "my village." Although the

intent may not be to imply ownership of a village, such language certainly has the tone of ownership. In light of the history of Native communities being imposed upon, particularly by non-Native outsiders, I find such language inappropriate and offensive. Rather, itinerant clinicians who travel to Native communities should refer to the Native village they work in by its name without any reference to "my village." It simply is a distraction. Such language, too, potentially can lead to a sense of ownership, a feeling of being identified or affiliated with a Native community, as if it is an object to be possessed. When we speak in a colonizing tone, we set in motion a wave that can create a reality where we "become" the language we use.

Psychological Testing and Diagnostic Labeling

The predation potential of psychological testing and diagnostic labeling is another colonizing pattern. In my two decades of working in the Bering Strait region, I have witnessed numerous youth sent to residential treatment facilities in Anchorage or other cities. Many times, youth undergo psychological testing to ascertain their strengths and weaknesses to help facilitate better treatment planning. I have observed such tests unfairly characterizing Native youth as mentally retarded when I know for a fact this is not the case. Often the Wechsler scales are used without any cross-validation of a more culturally fair intellectual test (e.g., Leiter International Performance Scale). Psychologists who are not sensitive to Native differences in learning style (i.e., nonverbal versus verbal learning) unfairly use the Full Scale IQ to characterize a child's general intellectual abilities when the difference between a Native youth's verbal versus nonverbal processing abilities is statistically significant. This has led to Native youth being perceived as intellectually deficient.

Given the relatively new *DSM-5*, however, standardized testing of intelligence when diagnosing intellectual disabilities must consider a child's level of adaptive functioning rather than IQ test scores alone. Without adequately considering adaptive functioning levels, a child's overall intellectual ability cannot be captured. The *DSM-5*'s removal of IQ test scores from the diagnostic criteria in favor of emphasizing severity of impairment based on adaptive functioning will, we hope, help minimize the unfair underestimation of Native youth intellectual ability. This is especially important in forensic cases, but it becomes magnified in the context of Alaska Native youth. Too, psychologists must be sensitive to acknowledging differences in a child's learning style when they have statistically significant differences between nonverbal and verbal comprehension abilities. In such circumstances, the Full Scale IQ cannot be used to provide an overall description of an individual's intellectual abilities. This seems to be common sense, yet using the Full Scale IQ when such differences exist continues to be a common practice.

Historically, psychiatry and mental healthcare in general have appeared to be in a hurry to pathologize people, leading many to question the validity of psychiatric diagnoses. The Rosenhan experiment (Rosenhan 1973; Morris 2018) famously demonstrates how psychiatric diagnoses can remain with a person even in light of evidence that contradicts such diagnoses. David Rosenhan, a psychologist and professor at Stanford University, conducted his study in two parts. The first part involved his sending healthy associates, including himself, to twelve psychiatric hospitals, where they feigned auditory hallucinations in order to gain admission. After being admitted, these pseudopatients behaved normally and told staff they were no longer hallucinating. The average time spent in these hospitals was nineteen days. Upon leaving, the pseudopatients had to admit to having a mental illness and agree to take prescribed antipsychotic medication. Further, all but one were diagnosed with schizophrenia in remission upon their release. (Interestingly, during their stay on the psychiatric units, the pseudopatients came under suspicion by thirty-five actual patients, who told staff that they thought the pseudopatients were not mentally ill.)

In the second part of Rosenhan's study, he was challenged by the staff of one teaching hospital to send them his pseudopatients. This hospital believed that their staff would not make the same error. Rosenhan agreed. The staff later maintained with confidence that they had identified forty-one of Rosenhan's pseudopatients from a total of 250 new patients who had been admitted to their facility. In fact, Rosenhan had not sent any pseudopatients to this teaching hospital.

Diagnostic labeling presents as a colonizing pattern because it can disempower an individual's strength and resiliency. As Saleebey (2006) maintains:

> Accentuating the problems of clients creates a wave of pessimistic expectations of, and predictions about, the client, the client's environment, and the client's capacity to cope with that environment. Furthermore, these labels have the insidious potential, repeated over time, to alter how individuals see themselves and how others see them. In the long run, these changes seep into the individual's identity. (4)

Our culture's fascination with problems and pathology is reflected in popular television programs like *The Jerry Springer Show*, among others. It is further fueled by the necessity of making a diagnosis for insurance purposes to ensure a rewarding business. This is not, however, to imply that diagnostic labeling is by itself harmful. But it underscores how labeling places mental health providers in a powerful position that can distance themselves from their clients by exercising power and control and, thereby, manipulating the relationship between the provider and those being helped. More importantly, it begs for exercising "balance to the equation of understanding and helping those who are hurting" (Saleebey 2006, 3). This balance, Saleebey elucidates, "requires that we appreciate the struggles of an individual, family, or community but that more importantly we look at those struggles for hints and intimations, or solid evidence of strengths, capacities, and competencies" (22).

When making a diagnosis, I habitually involve my clients by reading them the *DSM* criteria that appears to fit for their presenting problem. I have found that this process is empowering rather than disempowering, since it involves collaboration and an open atmosphere of trust while actively asking the client to acknowledge and explain symptoms. The power of the mental health provider is reduced. (I am reminded of one case involving a client for whom I could not come up with a diagnosis. I shared this openly with her. She, in turn, started talking about her anxiety issues and how she was previously diagnosed with anxiety. We subsequently explored criteria for anxiety and she was relieved that her problem was recognized and validated.) Further, I take a considerable amount of time to identify clients' strengths and to understand how they have successfully dealt with their presenting problem in the past. I emphasize the strengths people have for coping with their "pathology" rather than leaving them with a diagnosis that discourages them with pessimism and personal weakness, and potentially sends them on a path of self-fulfilling disappointment and failure.

Research

This is another area that can be laden with a colonizing flavor. At the time of this writing, I am on two research committees whose members are in large cities across the United States. While these committees are composed of well-intentioned individuals, I often wonder who benefits the most from them: the committee members or Alaska Natives? People of privilege or people who have been disempowered? I can proudly place my participation in these groups on my curriculum vitae. This looks impressive. It helps polish my professional presentation. Yet is this the real goal of my being on these committees that are theoretically intended to help Alaska Natives?

Tuhiwai Smith (1999), a Maori researcher, maintains that Western research is historically embedded in European imperialism and colonialism that promotes racism, ethnocentrism, and exploitation.

Mihesuah (1993), a Choctaw historian and writer, contends that researchers should not look upon American Indian/Alaska Native populations as curiosities; she suggests that those who conduct research on these peoples need to ask themselves why they are doing such research and ultimately who is benefiting.

Duran (2006) refers to researchers with a Western perspective entering Native communities as implementing "helicopter research": "Just as a helicopter touches down, takes off vertically, and disappears as if no one had ever been there, the researchers come and go, with few positive effects for the research 'subjects'" (113). He further maintains: "When the research is of a purely Western form, we have a neo-colonial activity being imposed on a community that is already suffering from historical trauma brought on by colonial processes" (114).

The Barrow Alcohol Study, undertaken in 1979, illustrates how researchers may abuse their power when working with cultures outside of their own. This study was intended to understand the relationship between alcohol and accidental death, suicide, and violence in rural Alaska. But it was conducted without adequate input from community members, and the researchers' measures were not valid for the people they were studying. Further, the results failed to consider factors grounded in culture, history, and politics. The findings were subsequently overgeneralized and made unfair and demeaning characterizations that were a tremendous insult to the people represented in the study (Foulks 1989; Wolf 1989).

To avoid the ethics violations and cultural insensitivities like those of the Barrow Alcohol Study, Native communities have begun to demand and embrace community-based participatory research (CBPR).[7] This approach is focused on a long-term commitment between researchers and community members to assess

---

7   I thank Dr. Jordan Lewis for educating me on community-based participatory research as well as his tremendous contributions to this particular field of research.

strengths, resources, and the needs of the community and to build local capacity.

The People Awakening Project (Allen and Mohatt 2014; Allen, Mohatt, Beehler and Rowe 2014; Allen, Mohatt, Fok, Henry, and Burkett 2014; Mohatt et al. 2014; Mohatt et al. 2004; Mohatt et al. 2007) represents a twenty-year partnership with Alaska Native communities using collaborative research methods. It was designed to study and promote healthy development in twelve-to-eighteen-year-old Alaska Native youth in rural Yup'ik communities. It identified factors on an individual, family, peer, and community level that protected against alcohol use. A long-term goal was to develop cultural interventions that reinforce and build upon such protective factors. Some of the findings underscored the importance of providing opportunities for youth involvement in the community, increasing support for youth within families, and teaching strategies for youth to embrace friends and family to solve problems and cope with stress. Suicide-prevention programs employing collaborative and strengths-based methods consistent with this study are being promoted in some Native communities within the Bering Strait region to date.

Community-based participatory research has also contributed to confronting inaccurate stereotypes of widespread alcohol abuse among Alaska Natives. In one research study, partially funded by the Norton Sound Economic Development Corporation (NSEDC), 134 Alaska Native Elders were interviewed in the Bering Strait region and Norton Sound. In the spirit of collaboration, university researchers worked with five Native communities over a two-year period, carefully interviewing Elders in their homes. The results of this study reflected very high rates of sobriety and low rates of alcohol use among Alaska Native Elders (Skewes and Lewis 2016).

The benefits of the People Awakening Project and CBPR appear to be growing and represent a shift to a positive focus on the strengths and resiliency of Alaska Natives and their communities.

Lewis and Allen (2017) examined motivating and maintenance factors for sobriety among older Alaska Native adults across Alaska. Their results illustrate how Alaska Native adults who quit drinking and maintain sobriety have a high regard for what has been defined as "indigenous cultural generativity": a high concern for and investment in caring for family and community, being a role model, and passing down their wisdom and experiences to younger generations. This research found that the central features promoting successful aging and sobriety in Alaska Native Elders were grounded in family, role expectations and socialization, and desire for community and culture engagement and spirituality.

I am involved in one Native village that has procured a grant from SAMHSA that is geared toward suicide prevention using the community readiness model (Plested, Jumper-Thurma, and Edwards 2016) and other culturally sensitive methods (see US Department of Health and Human Services 2010). This approach makes sense to me, since communities often have different levels of readiness for embracing solutions to preventing problems such as suicide. Further, it is sensitive to recognizing and adapting cultural solutions deemed appropriate by community members to the problems in their community.

Indigenous Community-Based Approaches to Solving Problems

Western clinical approaches have not always been well-received within Indigenous communities. Grassroots movements, developed locally by Native people, potentially provide a better "fit" for enhancing the emotional and behavioral well-being of Native people. This section describes grassroots Native approaches to solving problems. It is not exhaustive but is respectfully cognizant of community-based methods in Alaska Native communities. Two prominent grassroots programs within Alaska are highlighted here. These programs are consistent with supporting Native self-determination in that they are driven by local residents of Native villages solving their own problems.

Calricaraq

In one Native community, I participated in Calricaraq,[8] translated from Yup'ik as "Healthy Living," a three-day event sponsored by village leadership. Born from the wisdom of Yup'ik/Cup'ik Elders, Calricaraq showcases interactive and informational Indigenous approaches to recovering from impacts of historical and lifetime trauma, and it has been presented across the state. Participants learned how trauma has undermined Native culture and language, identity and spirituality, parenting skills, autonomy, and self-control—setting in motion generational patterns of dysfunctional and hurtful behavior that are still manifested today. Participants also learned about healing—finding meaning and significance in spite of the traumatic elements that plague Native individuals and communities. The use of hands-on, demonstrative exercises, rooted in traditional wisdom and knowledge, enhanced the learning of historical trauma and its effects on the body, mind, heart, and spirit. By reinforcing the traditional knowledge of Yup'ik/Cup'ik people, it reinforced the need for developing and teaching healthy coping skills. Participants engaged in both small and large group discussions that led to profound sharing of pain within a supportive atmosphere that instilled elements of hope and healing. Another positive aspect of Calricaraq is that it offers participants additional training so that they can implement this model within their own communities.

The Kake Peacemaking Circle

Implemented in 1998 by the Healing Heart Council, a group of concerned residents of Kake, the Kake Peacemaking Circle honored the

---

8   https://www.resourcebasket.org/calricaraq-training/

Craig Healing Totem. This totem was made by a grieving Tsimpsean wood carver, Stan Marsden, whose son died of a substance abuse overdose. Marsden's totem making was also made into a powerful film by Ellen Frankenstein, *Carved from the Heart* (New Day Films, 1997), and is a symbol of sobriety as well as healing from loss and trauma. Marsden made the totem to honor his son's memory. During its creation, the pole brought together the entire town of Craig, where community members faced the tragedy of loss on a healing journey characterized by mutual support, respect for culture, and art and ceremony. The film, too, acknowledges the generational grief within Alaska Native and American Indian communities stemming from the rapid changes in lifestyle and the disruption of Native traditions and knowledge.

The Kake Peacemaking Circle is a simple group process that can be easily taught by demonstration. The peacemaking circle process is used for suicide prevention, interventions for alcoholism, domestic violence, personal and cultural traumas, and restorative justice work. Peacemaking circles, built on values of loyalty, love, and compassion, are voluntary and open to everyone. Each circle creates its own ground rules that generally encompass respect, confidentiality, consensus, honesty, and caring. It recognizes that not every community is the same, and only the community can embrace strategies that work to improve health and strengthen community bonds. Peacemaking circles, therefore, are presented as potential mediums that can address a community's physical, psychological, social, and spiritual dimensions on a variety of health issues.

In Kake, the peacemaking circle meets twice a month. Those who elect to attend can sit in the circle as supporters or bring a problem for resolution. The circle also reaches out to community members who are perceived to be in need of help and support.

The first time the Kake Healing Heart Council held a circle, it was at the request of the Alaska Division of Family and Youth Services. That circle, and subsequent ones, supported a woman to stay sober from alcohol and resulted in her keeping custody of her children. The Kake magistrate has held eight restorative justice circles and follow-up circles for sixty residents. All are reported to have been a success.

In the context of restorative justice, peacemaking circles promote offender accountability and victim restoration. It is an alternative approach to criminal justice and court systems, allowing a group of people—including the offender, victim, and other community members—to respond to a particular crime or incident. Offenders receive support and supervision to promote positive change, while victims participate in developing sanctions and defining the elements that will remedy an injury perpetuated by an offender.

Many people from Kake have participated in the peacemaking circle, and many have commented on its benefit. Jada Smith explained:

> The circle has been a very powerful tool among our people, not just now but for generations. When we come together in a circle you can feel the power instantly. It's not just us sitting here. We represent our families, our fathers, our forefathers, our ancestors. It is such a privilege to work with our people. To love one another, to honor and respect each other enough so that we not only live for today, but our lives go on through our children and our grandchildren. The circle is a "living treasure" because it takes people who are alive and confident and powerful and concerned enough to come to the circle to make it work. It is hard to step out and do your part and talk from the heart, especially for our young people, to speak from the heart sincere words of compassion, love and concern. I know that it will be used for a long time because even now our children are using it. You can see into the future when you look at our children and it is a hopeful future—there's not one who's going to be defeated. We are not victims any longer. We are survivors.

Even gone past survivors. We are now empowered.
(Healthy Alaskans 2010, 8)

Important lessons learned from the Kake peacemaking circle experience that other communities may want to consider include:

- Communities can learn from each other
- Some solutions involve going back to traditional ways
- Improving community health is a long process that evolves in response to leadership, information available, community readiness and learning what works
- Listening, respect, compassion and trust are healing
- Individual healing heals communities
- A Circle is simple; training is available, you can do it
- Circles don't take money. (Healthy Alaskans 2010, 10)

A peacemaking circle embraces the spirit of people coming together to solve their own problems on their own terms. Once, in a Norton Sound village, I was asked to participate in a group meeting that had the tone of a circle. Two teenagers who historically had engaged in conflict with each other were voluntarily brought together, along with their parents, grandparents, and community Elders. People, including the teens, took turns sharing their perception of the problem. Solutions to the problem were then entertained. It was a very supportive process and resulted in the resolution of conflict between the teenagers. Although it was not a formal peacemaking circle, it nonetheless embodied some of its components of listening and respect. I am consistently amazed at the power of group meetings—whether it is group psychotherapy or talking circles—and their healing properties toward solving community and individual problems.

The Kake Peacemaking Circle has been implemented for over two decades. The method has been taught to and employed in other Alaska Native communities outside hub communities, including Juneau, Fairbanks, and Kenai (Alaska Court Magistrate Judge Mike Jackson, Organized Village of Kake, personal communication, 2019).[9]

Another outstanding resource is the book *Peacemaking Circles: From Conflict to Community* (Pranis, Stuart, and Wedge 2003), which explains the circle philosophy and its application to not only criminal justice issues but other areas of life involving hurts and conflicts within diverse community settings.

Tribal Problems, Tribal Solutions

The Office of the Attorney General, Department of Justice, issued guidelines articulating principles for working with federally recognized Native tribes. One overarching principle asserted:

> The Department of Justice is committed to tribal self-determination, tribal autonomy, tribal nation-building, and the long-term goal of maximizing tribal control over governmental institutions in tribal communities, because tribal problems generally are best addressed by tribal solutions, including solutions informed by tribal traditions and custom. (*Federal Register* 2014, 1)

In a similar spirit, Napoleon (1996, 30) reminds us:

> it is a mistake to think that Congress or any other group can bring the Alaska Native people back to health. Money, programs, or loans, no matter how well intentioned, cannot end the unhappiness, dissatisfaction,

---

9   More information can be found at: www.kake-nsn.gov.

anger, frustration, and sorrow that is now leading so
many Alaska Natives to alcohol abuse, alcoholism, and
tragedy. Only Alaska Natives can do this. To look else-
where for solutions is illusory.

The above underscores the importance of non-Native and Native
mental health providers being sensitive to Native self-determination
and the colonization processes that have undermined it. Duran
(2006) stresses the importance of Native communities being aware
of their history and the trauma that has contributed to present-day
problems. He maintains: "Consciousness raising and specific interventions dealing with historical trauma and internalized oppression
should be part of an overall community healing process" (118).

Non-Native mental health providers cannot solve Native community problems. But we can support and participate in village-based
efforts toward this goal. And, within the context of working with our
individual Native clients, we can promote consciousness-raising and
prosocial behaviors to deal with trauma and internalized oppression.

Personal Biases/Worldview

Considering our clients' worldview is vital to understanding them
and the context they live in. Without such sensitivity, we may be
prone to unnecessary personal biases permeating our work.

In my first year in the Bering Strait region, I was invited by Rural
Cap to observe a Head Start classroom within a very traditional village, where the children still spoke their Native language. On a cold
winter morning, I entered the preschool, selecting a quiet corner
to sit and observe without intruding (or so I had thought) as three-
to-four-year-old children entered their classroom bundled in heavy
winter parkas.

I watched as the boys and girls followed their morning routine of
hanging up their hats and coats before having free play. Breakfast

was soon served, and the children eagerly took their seats along with their teachers to receive the morning meal.

More children arrived. I noticed one girl clinging to her mother by the coatracks. She appeared to be observing me with fear in her eyes, crying, as her mother tried to comfort her while coaxing her out of her parka.

Separation anxiety, I immediately thought. The girl was about four years old, and she was probably having problems leaving her mother and her familiar home in lieu of immersing herself in her expanding world of Head Start.

Not an unusual problem for a preschooler, I further ventured. Leaving the comfort of home and attending preschool can be terrifying for some kids and is not a reflection of poor parenting but underscores an important developmental milestone for young children.

I continued observing intermittently the tearful girl and her mother, who appeared increasingly uncomfortable. If I were to work with this child, I reasoned, I would spend most of my time with the girl's mother. First, I would explain to the mother the phenomenon of separation anxiety and how it is a normal behavior and not a reflection of her daughter being emotionally disturbed. Often, when parents bring their children to see me they are consumed with guilt—thinking that their children's problems are a sure sign that they are doing something wrong as parents when, in fact, children frequently have problems that are a natural progression of their development. Second, I would enlist the mother's support in developing a game plan to help her daughter's growing independence and autonomy. We would meet with the Head Start teachers and create a timeline illustrating the different hours of the day in colors so that the child would know when her mother would return to pick her up at the end of the day. Further, I might suggest that the mother provide her daughter with a transitional object, such as a picture of mother and daughter together. This would give the girl a sense of security she could hold on to throughout the day. I would also give the mother instructions to reassure her daughter that she would return without fail when school was over. Finally, I would tell her to promptly leave the classroom after saying her goodbyes and let her daughter's teachers deal with the girl's fears, since her mother's continued presence only served to reinforce the child's clinginess and insecurities.

While talking with the Head Start director, I casually commented that the little girl by the coatracks seemed to be having separation anxiety with her mother. The director looked at me with a puzzled expression. She then bluntly commented: "She doesn't have separation anxiety. She's just afraid of white people."

My morning lesson at Head Start was over.

My experience illustrates how easily a non-Native mental health professional can superimpose Western views of psychology on a culture they may have little understanding of and/or experience with. In retrospect, I retained a mindset that was prematurely and unfairly superimposed on a culture whose norms I was not sensitive to. I engaged in a colonizing mindset and repeated the crime of oppression Native people have historically experienced since I was operating within a culturally insensitive and inaccurate dogma. The way I saw the problem *was* the problem.

The mother who huddled uncomfortably beside her tearful daughter was doing exactly what any good parent should have been doing: protecting her child from a perceived danger. I had judged her unfairly. When I conceptualized the problem as separation anxiety, I had entirely missed the point because I did not take the time to understand.

Instead, I had become the problem.

As non-Native and Native mental health professionals working within Native communities, we need to practice walking softly with our Westernized mindsets held in suspension. We need to make a concerted effort to understand the people and the culture we work with, or else we make things potentially worse for Alaska Natives.

Alaska Natives have legitimate ways of knowing and conceptualizing reality. It is imperative that mental health professionals genuinely seek to understand them and their culture. Elders have repeatedly told me that outsiders need to be careful not to impose their Western worldview on Native people and their communities. At an Elder lunch one day, one woman explained that she becomes upset when she hears the local radio station interview Western professionals on medical or mental health problems. She told me that she often wants to call in and tell the radio station not to forget that the views being discussed come from a Western worldview—not a Native worldview. To practice culturally competent care with our Native clients, we must be mindful of the worldviews we harbor that might be inappropriately superimposed on our Native clients. Conversely, we must be sensitive, mindful, and eager to learn the worldviews of our Native clients.

Generalist Orientation

For mental health professionals working in rural Alaska Native communities, a generalist orientation is vital. Mental health providers need to be comfortable working with all ages, from preschool to the elderly, and with all types of presenting problems. For those therapists who lack training with a certain population, acquiring such training under the supervision of a qualified colleague is essential. Training is also essential for those who are uncomfortable with certain presenting problems. Many therapists, for example, prefer not to see substance abuse clients. Yet to not accept these clients is potentially unethical. Further, many people suffering from substance abuse also suffer from emotional problems and vice versa. To focus exclusively on one problem compromises the other. Creating a dichotomy between mental health and substance abuse is a disservice to clients and disempowers the people we intend to help. Mental health care should automatically assume that substance abuse is a part of such services. This is not a novel concept. It is, for example, consistent with mental health care services followed by the Veterans Administration.

Hurting Helpers

As mental health providers, we often work with clients struggling with codependent issues. Codependence is "any suffering and/or dysfunction that is associated with or results from focusing on the needs and behavior of others" (Whitfield 2006, 28). The codependent individual is so focused on and preoccupied with the needs of others that they neglect their own needs. The needs and lives of codependent people become secondary to those of others surrounding them. The field of self-awareness is obscured, filled only with focus on others.

Whitfield (2006) succinctly describes the growth of codependence:

1. Invalidation and repression of internal cues, such as our observations, feelings and reactions.
2. Neglecting our needs.
3. Beginning to stifle our Child Within.
4. Denial of a family or other secret.
5. Increasing tolerance of and numbness to emotional pain.
6. Inability to grieve a loss to completion.
7. Blocking of growth (mental, emotional, spiritual).
8. Compulsive behaviors in order to lessen pain and to glimpse our Child Within.
9. Progressive shame and loss of self-esteem.
10. Feeling out of control. Need to control more.
11. Delusion and projection of pain.
12. Stress-related illness develops.
13. Compulsion worsens.
14. Progressive deterioration:
    - Extreme mood swings.
    - Difficulty with intimate relationships.
    - Chronic unhappiness.
    - Interference with recovery from alcoholism/ CD and other conditions. (30–31)

While codependency can be a prominent issue with our clients, it also presents as a poignant problem with many people in the helping professions. I recall working with a medical provider in Wisconsin who worked tirelessly in her job as a frontline emergency responder. She sacrificed her own needs to such a severe degree that over many years her body began to suffer from stress-related ailments and conditions. Attempts to teach her relaxation methods were initially futile. She would not allow herself to relax because, as she phrased it, it made her feel "out of control." Her history, as she eventually began to convey and put into words, was laden with childhood sexual abuse. It was only after she began a journey of narrating and giving form to the secret trauma she had suffered that she gradually learned to relax, acknowledge some of her needs, and enjoy life.

In the mental health profession, understanding our motives and core beliefs for helping others is essential. Being sensitive to our own needs while helping others makes us better-grounded mental health providers who exercise healthy boundaries with our clients and with ourselves. Working in a rural Native community, where issues of self-determination and dependency abound, healthy boundaries are crucial (see Figure 3).

Some motivations underlying people working in the helping professions include:

- The lust for power (the need to have a sense of control with our surroundings while working with people who appear worse off than ourselves)
- Meeting our own needs (needing our clients to be needful to bolster our own self-esteem)
- The need to be liked (to be seen as a helper, a good person, to ingratiate our own sense of self-worth)
- The wish to heal. (Hawkins and Shohet 2012, 28–32)

The aforementioned motivations for pursuing work in the helping professions appear, at face value, self-serving and hedonistic. Yet they are negative only to the extent that such motivations remain outside a helper's field of awareness. As Hawkins and Shohet (2012) eloquently explain: "It is only the denial of needs that makes them dangerous. It is knowing ourselves and our motives that makes us more likely to be of real help. In that way we do not use others unawarely, for our own ends, or project parts of ourselves we cannot face onto our clients" (31).

Personal Well-Being (PWB)

Although identifying the dynamics contributing to a Native client's presenting problem is important, identifying the forces that make the client resilient to mental health problems is equally valuable. Understanding how Native clients describe personal wellness can serve as a referent for treatment goals and for monitoring treatment progress. Reimer's (1999) work, emphasizing personal well-being (PWB), with Iñupiat Natives found many descriptions that clients used to denote a personal state of wellness. While older people, for example, tended to use the words *ahregah* ("that's fine") or *nagooruk* ("feel good"), youth preferred words such as *well-being, feeling good, wellness*, and *healthy and whole* (6).

The Yup'ik word for not feeling well is *arrah*, while *assirrtuk* refers to feeling well, feeling good. Native individuals have shared that activities that promote a sense of feeling well or feeling good are caring and doing something with family; being involved in community events; doing traditional activities such as dancing; and practicing traditional values such as helping others. Strong social networks, including relationships with family, peers, and community members, and learning and practicing traditional activities and subsistence activities have been identified as protective factors and causal forces that enhance the mental health of Indigenous circumpolar youth (DeCou, Skewes, and Lopez 2013; MacDonald et al. 2013; MacDonald et al. 2015; Wexler et al. 2016).

Asking your client what word they prefer to call a personal state of wellness can be useful. During her research on PWB, some of Reimer's (2002) interview questions were: What makes you happy and feeling good? What takes away happiness and feeling good? In the spirit of Viktor Frankl (1959), I also like to expand upon Reimer's questions and ask, "What gives meaning to your life?" Invariably, many Native clients identify their relationships with family as being vital to providing them with a sense of purpose and meaning in life.

I once worked with a young Native woman who had been separated from her children for a number of reasons. She had become so distraught she was suicidal. We explored her situation—considering the forces that led to her being separated from her children and her options for reuniting with them. She concluded that her situation was not permanent, and that she was not destined to live her life separate from her children. Yet, as we considered the option of suicide, she realized that killing herself would be a permanent solution to a temporary circumstance. Further, we explored collaboratively how killing herself would affect her children.

This led her to become distraught and angry at several relatives whom she was close to and who had committed suicide. I gently explored with her that, similarly, this would be the residual emotional impact on her children if she chose to kill herself, and the potential for her own children to choose suicide in the future might increase. We concluded that she had the opportunity to stop the intergenerational transmission of suicide by being a responsible role model to her children. And, although being separated from her children was certainly a significant stressor, she had options to exercise to reunite with them. The bottom line: she was not helpless; she had ways to move her life in a proactive direction.

Further, I have found that augmenting questions of personal health and happiness with Berg and de Shazer's (1994) scaling questions can be a useful gauge for quantifying a client's personal state of wellness as well as a helpful therapeutic tool. Giving a client the opportunity to provide a narrative to scaling scores as to how they are maintaining this state is also useful. For example, a mental health provider might ask: "Given a scale of 0 to 10, with 10 being the highest, what score would you give your PWB (or the word the client prefers to use for personal wellness) this week?" If the score is lower than 10, a provider might ask: "What would make it a 10?" Other questions: "What factors are making your score lower than a 10?" "What factors might increase your score?"

Scaling questions can be applied to many areas of functioning in life (see, for example, Droby 2000).

Native Spirituality

For Native individuals in Alaska, spirituality is interwoven with the concept of personal well-being (Reimer 1999). To talk about one invariably leads to acknowledging the other. Alaska Native spirituality has been linked to a relationship with the land and traditional values and practices (Fienup-Riordan 1990), and Native American spirituality in general has been inextricably joined to a reverence for the earth and Indigenous rituals. The influence of European colonialism and imperialism, and the defacing of the world and the destruction of the natural environment, has been seen as a direct assault on Native American spirituality (Versluis 1992). The destruction of earth is seen as wounding its soul and the souls of the human beings who live on unhealed land (Duran 2006).

A White husband of an Iñupiat woman commented, "My wife is most alive, happy, when she is doing her traditional Native activities." Others have observed that they feel at their best when immersed in traditional rituals of dance and subsistence activities. Connection to traditional values and cultural roots is seen as a source of significant healing, so much so that one Yup'ik woman left a good-paying job in Anchorage to return to her Native village (*Alaska Dispatch*

News, January 9, 2016). The importance of being attuned to a Native client's spirituality and personal state of well-being can have potential implications for suicide risk and use of alcohol (Reimer 2002).

I have observed that many Yup'ik and Iñupiat clients tell of visitations from the spirit world. The most common appear to be dreams where a person's dead relatives or others "visit" them. One client explained that she had a dream in which she knew that it was her father, although she had never seen him since he died shortly after she was born. This had occurred twice over the course of several years, and this individual finally told her mother, who became tearful as she heard her daughter speak of the man in her dreams who fit the description of her past husband perfectly.

Other visitations come in the form of olfactory sensations. One young woman who tragically died habitually took saunas with her mother along with her relatives and friends. After she died, her mother and others were taking a sauna one evening and the distinct scent of rose suddenly filled the *mukaq* house (sauna house). Rose had been the deceased daughter's favorite soap and shampoo. The mother initially noticed the smell, and then others taking a sauna commented on smelling the fragrance as well. "It was my daughter visiting," the mother explained.

Tactile visitations are also common. One Native individual, while sleeping in a hotel in Anchorage, was repeatedly awoken by the gentle caress of someone tickling her toes and feet. She thought it was her husband, but upon waking she saw that he was sleeping soundly. The touching continued on other nights throughout the week. On one occasion, it progressed to her legs being forcefully held down on her bed so she could not get up. In Yup'ik culture, an interpretation of such a phenomenon foretells of something bad in the future. The touching that began with gentle caresses but then progressed to forceful possession, therefore, became a frightening event for this woman.

The actual witnessing of spiritual phenomenon constitutes another form of visitation. One individual told of seeing her father's spirit in her home. It was a comforting presence, something she was not afraid of but rather welcomed.

Many Native clients experience premonitions of something bad about to happen. One commented about her uncomfortable feelings: "I feel scared because I don't know what's going to happen. I have dreams, too, of people who have died, and then I know someone will die but I don't know who. I've been told by Elders that it's a special gift but I don't like it."

Melvin Riley, one of the first military men recruited into the army's psychic research program, maintains that Native Americans have always appreciated spiritual phenomenon but only recently has Western society seriously considered it. He explains that remote viewing (the Western technical term for such phenomenon) is the acquisition of any type of information (other than that experienced through the five senses) that emerges regardless of distance or time; it is an extension of our five senses, and it is an ongoing, everyday experience for every human being. Some people, however, are better receptors than others.

Riley, an accomplished remote viewer himself, mentored several military officers using this ability to locate hidden enemy military assets. He has appeared in numerous books and documentaries on remote viewing (Marrs 1997; Moorehouse 1996; Schnabel 1997; Wall to Wall Television 1995). He explains that remote viewing has always been known by Native Americans. The seminal book *Black Elk Speaks* (Neihardt 1932), for example, is a reflection of remote viewing. Further, Native American tribes employed this practice long before European influence. Tribes used remote viewers as a method to protect their people from attacks or as a way to find lost objects or companions. Today, many Native Americans still possess the powerful ability of remote viewing. However, because European influences have taught them to disown such traditional attributes, many Natives—particularly the younger generation are uncomfortable with their unique abilities. Many, Riley contends, are afraid of these special skills because they have not been educated regarding their valid existence and their use (Riley, personal communication, 1999).

Native Identity

Native peoples in the western hemisphere came heavily in contact with Europeans in the sixteenth and seventeenth centuries. Initially, Europeans benefited from Native people's knowledge of clothing, transportation, and hunting methods, but later on Native peoples assumed many features of European life, particularly those traits imposed by colonial governments, missionaries, and teachers. *Acculturation* refers to mutual changes that occur on a population level between cultures, involving ecological, cultural, social, and institutional factors, whereas changes that occur within individuals—involving behavior, identity, values, and attitudes—are referred to as *psychological acculturation* (Berry 1990). I have found the work of Berry and his colleagues useful when considering Alaska Native identity in the context of psychological acculturation and post-European contact. Further, there are many possible responses to this process. Just as communities deal with acculturative influences in a varied manner, individuals also adjust in a diverse fashion.

In their framework encompassing the psychology of acculturation, Berry, Trimble, and Olmeda (1986) describe how the mutual process of a dominant group and the acculturating group incur changes at the population and individual levels. The dominant culture (Culture A) exerts a stronger influence on the less dominant culture (Culture B) and its individuals (Individual B), although the dominant culture can incur changes too (e.g., population expansion, cultural diversification, governmental policy changes involving immigration). Culture B's influence on Individual B is "enculturation," a process of socializing the person to his/her Indigenous culture.

In this acculturation process, individuals can adopt various identities, attitudes, and behaviors (Berry et al. 1989). Some individuals may choose an assimilation option whereby they give up their Indigenous identity associated with Culture B and instead embrace the attitudes and behaviors of Culture A. Others may choose a separatist choice where they maintain their identity and behaviors aligned with Culture B while rejecting those of Culture A. Still other individuals may choose not to align themselves with either culture. Finally, other individuals may choose an integrative or bicultural option where they maintain their identity and many cultural practices of their Indigenous culture (Culture B) but simultaneously identify with the attitudes and behaviors aligned with Culture A; these individuals can move seamlessly between either culture. Berry (1997, 2005) contends that the integration strategy produces the most positive adaptation for individuals in the acculturation process.

Another aspect of the acculturation process involves the stress incurred by individuals immersed in it. Some authors refer to this as "culture shock" (Winkelman 1994). Berry (1990) describes the consequences of acculturated stress as involving "societal disintegration and personal crisis" whereby "the old social order and cultural norms often disappear, and individuals may be lost in the change" (246). He explains further:

> There is often a particular set of stress behaviors that occur during acculturation, such as lowered mental health status (especially confusion, anxiety, depression), feelings of marginality and alienation, heightened psychosomatic symptom level, and identity confusion. Acculturative stress is thus a phenomenon that may underlie a reduction in the health status of individuals (including physical, psychological, and social aspects). (246–247)

Working with Alaska Natives, I have seen that the phenomenon of acculturated stress is real and its consequences are palpable. In a study by the Alaska State Department of Health and Social Services analyzing completed suicides between 2003 and 2008, identity

confusion was cited as one dynamic contributing to the self-inflict-
ed deaths of Alaska Native men between the ages of twenty and
twenty-nine—at a rate thirteen times higher than the national rate.
Young Alaska Native men and women leaving their village and going
to college in larger cities such as Anchorage or Fairbanks presents
as another potential stress. I have observed this transition to be positive for some Alaska Natives and negative for others. In one circumstance, a Native woman could not cope with the stress of living
apart from her village and family, and returned to her village just a
few months after her first semester at college. In another example,
a young Native woman successfully completed her degree and returned to her village to become a political leader in her community.
Other individuals who have similarly received a degree or certification in some skill have returned to their village only to experience
being shamed by their peers, as if their going outside to gain a skill
meant forsaking their culture and community. However, with others
who have acquired a degree and/or vocational skill, I have witnessed
their families and friends proudly embracing their accomplishments.

Alaska Natives attending college or moving to cities such as
Anchorage have shared what they have found helpful in this process.
Alaska Natives moving out of the village to attend college consistently cite the support offered by their educational institution as vital
for coping with the stress involved in this transition. In particular, a
supportive professor or teacher is recognized as crucial to their success. This positive relational dynamic is an important foundation for
coping. Additionally, having a group of friends to associate with on
a daily basis and who are experiencing similar stress is also observed
to be integral to successful coping. One Alaska Native student found
that making friends among other minority groups (e.g., Asian) who
shared similar acculturative stress was important in her transition to
college life and also to life in the dominant culture in general.

Simply moving to a hub community such as Nome can also
be stressful. Many Alaska Natives living in the villages try to live

in Nome due to more employment opportunities. In this process, they also experience acculturative stress grounded in leaving their friends, family, and community and entering a society where some experience being marginalized and not socially accepted. One Alaska Native man, for example, shared his feelings of being discriminated against and mistreated.

The pressures that some Alaska Natives experience in the acculturation equation are real. Alaska Natives who are considering a move to acquire more education and/or a skill can present with significant concomitant acculturative stress. Recognizing this stress within the context of mental health treatment, and considering ways to successfully negotiate it, can be helpful.

The Assets Study

In 1990, Search Institute (www.search-institute.org) released a framework of developmental assets that contribute to prosocial behavior in youth across home, school, and community settings. External assets that instill support, boundaries, and structured time use, coupled with internal assets that instill educational commitment, positive values, and social competencies, were identified through data collected from over half a million seventh- through twelfth-graders throughout the Lower 48. Search's research found that the more assets youth had, the less likely they were to engage in problematic behaviors such as alcohol and other drugs, early sexual activity, depression/suicide, and antisocial behaviors such as violence, and the more likely they were to demonstrate school success and caring behaviors such as volunteering (Benson, Galbraith, and Espeland 1995).

The study was replicated with youth from Alaska and Canada (Association of Alaska School Boards 1998, Association of Alaska School Boards' Alaska Initiative for Community Engagement 2003).

Of forty assets identified, only 9 percent of Alaska youth surveyed had at least thirty-one. Key components of the asset framework were: helping children and teenagers develop good relationships is vital to their future development; all children and teenagers can use more assets than they have now; from infancy through adulthood, the process of building and enhancing assets for youth is ongoing; no single asset is the key to a child's positive future development; everyone has a role to play in a child's development; and small things count and it can be simply acknowledging a child by his/her name that can provide an important moment of support in that child's day (Association of Alaska School Boards 1998).

One Elder in Kake described the forty assets as: "This is so simple! All it is is 40 words that describe love" (Association of Alaska School Boards 1998, 13).

When I present the developmental assets framework, I emulate its delivery in the manner it was taught to me years ago. After I explain the Search Institute's research, workshop participants form a circle. Using a ball of yarn, I identify one asset that helps youth promote positive behavior (this is usually an asset I do with my own children to make it more personal). I then toss the ball of yarn across the circle to a person on the other side, who then also identifies an asset that promotes positive behavior. This is repeatedly done until a web is created across the circle. When a web starts to develop, I then have a group participant toss two balloons (which were blown up prior to this activity) into the web of yarn. Each balloon symbolizes a child. If enough assets were identified, the web should catch the "child." If the balloon falls through, the group counts the number of assets that were created. This number typically is low (e.g., twelve), which parallels the process that if not enough assets are created for a child, they may "fall" through the web and become hurt in some manner (e.g., using drugs).

Additionally, asset checklists can be provided to parents so that they can perform their own gauge of how well they are creating assets for their children. This can provide feedback on what areas they may focus on in the future to enhance their children's assets and those of youth in their community as well.

The assets framework can be a nice addition to a parenting workshop that includes the previously discussed parent-child interaction therapy. It is an "upstream" approach that is easy to use and proactive. Further, the developmental assets profile (DAP), based on the eight categories of developmental assets, has been effectively used as a measurement tool and adapted to study and promote positive youth development in other cultural settings (Romano 2015; Scales 2011; Scales et al. 2013).

Flow

Flow is a term coined by Csikszentmihalyi (1990) that can be brought into a client's therapy since it can enhance self-esteem and overall well-being. Specifically, it involves a rewarding experience in which a person is totally absorbed in what they are doing, paying attention to implementing a task to the point that they are unaware of outside stimuli. Optimal states of flow occur when an individual's skill level is delicately balanced with the difficulty level of the task at hand. That is, the task should ideally challenge the person's skill level to the degree that the activity is challenging but does not produce overwhelming anxiety; conversely, the flow activity should be interesting to the individual and not so overly easy as to render boredom.

The practice of flow can be found in many activities within a Native community such as subsistence activities, Native dancing, sewing, beading, and non-Native activities such as basketball and cross-country skiing. Within the context of therapy, flow can help validate the usefulness and purpose of such activities and reinforce their relevance—bringing them into the fold of self-regulatory methods that enhance our sense of wellness.

Tribal Healers

In our eagerness to practice Western ways of mental health treatment, we must not forget the traditional healers of Alaska Native communities. We must not minimize their importance to providing culturally relevant care. We must not replicate the Christian missionary movement that misunderstood traditional healers: "Missionaries portrayed all types of traditional healers simplistically as evil, when in reality, our healers were tribal members who followed specific clan protocols regarded as sacred. When missionaries condemned and banned the practices of our community healers and medicine persons, our methods to keep peace and balance in our communities were devalued; they ceased in some areas and became less common in other areas. We recognize that many indigenous cultures have medicine people still ingrained in their midst" (Alaska Native Tribal Health Consortium 2014, 14).

The Norton Sound Health Corporation has recently added a section to our behavioral health assessment form asking if a client is accessing traditional healers. I have accessed traditional healers for my own problems. Likewise, we should be mindful to let our clients know that traditional healers are available to promote healing and balance in their bodies and in their lives.

Learning and Communication Styles

As mental health providers, particularly non-Native ones, it is prudent to remember that our Native clients do not always conform to assimilating and processing information within the verbal modality that is often emphasized in the Western culture. I once worked with a Native woman who was noncommunicative. Instead of judging her as "resistant" or "noncompliant," I engaged her in the use of scaling questions (see "Strengths Perspective"). On a piece of paper, I drew the scale of 0 to 10 and explained that 10 indicated her doing well and 0 meant she was not doing well; and of course in between 0 and 10 reflected various degrees of wellness. Through this visual medium, she was able to rate her degree of wellness. Further, I had her write down those elements or factors that supported her score. After this was completed, and because her score was lower than a 10, I circled the number 10 and asked her to identify those factors that would make her a 10 today. She was able to do this as well. Through this medium, the quiet Native woman provided me with a rich source of information that was helpful in my work with her.

The learning and communication styles of Native individuals is prefaced with the following three elements (Pewewardy 2002; Swisher 1990):

- Native learning styles should not be categorized into one specific or absolute learning style;
- Although research may describe specific patterns of learning among some American Indian/Alaska Native groups, there are significant differences among tribes and the individuals within them; and
- Differences, diversity, in learning styles is common among all cultures (Pewewardy, 2002; Swisher, 1990).

Given the above qualifiers, we must keep them in mind when reviewing some research support for:

- The view that American Indians/Alaska Native individuals are visual learners;
- The view that American Indians/Alaska Native individuals learn best when they are able to see the material they are expected to master;
- The view that American Indians/Alaska Native individuals learn best when they are provided a myriad of visual learning opportunities such as graphs, films, demonstrations and pictures; and

- The view that American Indians/Alaska Native individuals learn best when presented with the bigger picture first, using a holistic strategy, rather than building upon a concept via details first (Pewewardy 2002).

Being mindful of our clients' learning styles helps facilitate a better therapeutic relationship that offers increased communication and mutual understanding.

Maslow's Hierarchy of Needs

A father in tears because he cannot provide enough food for his family. Subzero temperatures, the heating oil has run out, and the money to pay for another fifty gallons of oil has also run out. Children wrapping their own toys in newspaper and placing them under the Christmas tree because their parents do not have enough money to buy gifts. A young man demoralized, in a perpetual state of malaise, because he cannot find a job. Families displaced for lack of shelter. Community members and community leaders worried over the high rate of cancer among their people and pondering the residual effects of past military installations on their land and on the animals and plants they depend on for subsistence.

These are but a few scenarios met in rural Alaska villages. Maslow's hierarchy of needs reminds mental health providers working in rural communities that sometimes basic physiological needs such as food and shelter and basic safety needs such as financial security, health and well-being, overall personal security, and protection from adverse impacts of external factors beyond their control take precedence over a fifty-minute therapy hour.

Maslow's hierarchy of needs is not entirely applicable to Native communities, due to its emphasis on the needs and drives of an individualistic society that focuses on self-improvement, with self-actualization being at the pinnacle of self-improvement, in lieu of collectivistic societies where the needs of acceptance and community outweigh the needs for freedom and individuality. And yet its recognition of lower-order needs (i.e., physiological and safety) remind mental health providers not to get lost doing simple counseling when a client's basic needs are being denied. Case management may be needed.

For example, one mother became tearful in session and shared her frustration and grief at her inability to feed her family, particularly toward the end of the month when money ran out. She talked about how she does not qualify for the community food bank. A phone call to the ICWA worker in charge of the community food bank said that the woman's perception was wrong—that while she did not qualify for another community resource, she most certainly qualified for the food bank. The woman had mistakenly believed that the one resource she was *not* eligible for disqualified her from the other resource. With this perception cleared up, the woman felt relief that she could seek support for her family with the community food bank.

Trust/Mistrust

It takes time for a Native community to develop trust with an outsider, particularly a non-Native professional in the field of mental health, who may not be readily accepted as a source of help. In my experience, trust begins to develop after a year in a Native village; two to three years helps add to this process. I recall going on vacation at the beginning of my second year in one village. When I returned, some people remarked, "You came back?" Other people asked, "Do you like living here?"

The high turnover rate among mental health clinicians in Alaska in general does not help develop trust. Stable, committed mental health workers in rural Alaska appear to be a persistent need. In an overview of mental health services for American Indians and Alaska

Natives in the 1990s, the Indian Health Service of the US Public Health Service concluded:

> The geographic isolation and harsh climatic conditions of some tribal locations create difficult problems of adaptation for some professional staff, particularly those who are non-Native and who have little or no experience with Native Americans. The high demand for services in many mental health programs, combined with the complexity and seriousness of mental health needs and the occasional lack of support from other health program personnel or tribal members frequently results in high rates of burnout and turnover among mental health professionals. (Nelson et al. 1992, 259)

The stigma associated with mental health problems is another significant dynamic contributing to the mistrust toward mental health providers. One client commented: "People are too proud to admit to any personal problems. Showing your vulnerability is not encouraged. Also, in my culture we have a value toward avoiding conflict." Interestingly, the self-stigma that this client expressed has been associated with more negative help-seeking attitudes among some Alaska Natives (see, for example, Freitas-Murrell and Swift 2015).

Exploring the meaning of "mental illness" and its various forms of expression with clients can help destigmatize mental health services (Grandbois 2005). I have had several clients tell me that my humanizing and normalizing their personal problems helped them overcome their initial reluctance and embarrassment toward seeing me. Some had delayed making contact due to fears of being perceived as a "nutcase" or being diagnosed as mentally disturbed, suitable for long-term internment in a psychiatric hospital.

Stigma around mental health issues is not a Native phenomenon but appears worldwide. For example, Meghan Markle and Prince Harry are planning to launch a show with Oprah Winfrey focusing on mental health (Gonzales 2019). Prince Harry, who has shared his own experiences and is an advocate for ending stigma around mental health issues, also founded the mental well-being campaign Heads Together with Prince William and Kate Middleton.

Working with Schools in Alaska Native Communities

I have had wonderful working relationships with school personnel in Alaska Native communities, and I have had horrible working relationships with school personnel in Alaska Native communities. Mutual respect of boundaries appears integral to honing a viable working relationship between a mental health provider employed by the local tribal health corporation and a teacher and/or principal employed by the state.

Although psychologists can do much (or more) of the testing done by a school psychologist, for example, a school may want their own personnel doing such testing. We must respect that, although we may offer some input to a school, particularly if we are approached by parents to do testing/assessment on their children.

I have witnessed itinerant clinicians coming into a Native community and spending an entire day—at the request of school personnel—counseling students without parental consent. We must resist the temptation, too, of being called into a classroom to do behavioral management on a student going ballistic because they cannot master the new math material. Schools must follow their own protocols (e.g., calling in the local village police officer) for managing the behavior of disruptive students, particularly those presenting with issues grounded in danger to self and/or others, although the itinerant clinician can certainly assist in these difficult circumstances. I remember one school principal calling me and screaming for me to come to the school to counsel a student who was out of control. I instead instructed the principal to call the student's parent to come get them and bring them to my office, where I would gladly meet with the student.

Depending on the receptivity of a school's administration, many village-based behavioral health aides/practitioners make regular weekly visits to schools to present on topics ranging from managing anger in prosocial ways to positive problem-solving. I have often been a part of these presentations, which are fun and meaningful to the youth in a Native community. Further, involving Elders in these presentations adds depth, making them more productive and culturally relevant.

Ethics

Mental health providers working in rural areas face unique challenges (Schank 1998). Living and working in a small community, where people are familiar with one another, invariably invites conflict. Potential boundary issues easily arise. The nature of our profession, too, may place us in uncomfortable situations where we need to exercise ethical decisions that lead to conflict with other community members. On another level, what will you do when the ethical principles governing the mental health profession conflict with the law?

We must "do the right thing" nonetheless. Ethics are not optional.

Psychological Testing and Alaska Natives

Psychological assessment in American Indian and Alaska Native communities has been plagued with culturally inappropriate services and test interpretation (Allen 2002). In this section I share what has worked for me with regard to some psychological testing with Alaska Natives. It is not an exhaustive review: I do not cover all psychological tests I have used, but I do describe the main ones I regularly employ. The psychological tests I identify here have, I believe, successfully addressed referral questions I have received over the past two decades in a culturally sensitive manner. I cite empirical support for the instruments I use where there is such support. What follows is my clinical experience with testing and my attempt to make it as culturally relevant as possible for the Alaska Natives I work with. I believe that these have been helpful, not harmful, to the Alaska Natives I have tested.

Although this section comments on specific tests, I want to emphasize that they do not replace common sense and sound clinical judgment. For example, if a student has not been in school for many months due to sickness or an unstable home environment, any intellectual assessment must be done with extraordinary caution so that an individual is not unfairly labeled. Also, when assessing for problems such as ADHD, a sound clinical interview is necessary to rule out factors that may be causing a child to be overly active (e.g., abuse, exposure to domestic violence, etc.). In short, a psychological test must not be used in isolation from other sources of information.

Intellectual Functioning

I have used the Wechsler scales (from the Psychological Corporation) with all ages of Alaska Natives. There are two important ways to make these tests more culturally sensitive:

1. Because sometimes there is a significant difference between an Alaska Native's nonverbal and verbal comprehension skills, an examiner must interpret the difference between these two abilities. As previously mentioned, I have read reports from psychologists who have given the Wechsler to Alaska Natives and who interpret the Full Scale IQ when there is a statistically significant difference between Verbal Comprehension and Perceptual Reasoning indices. This simply does not make sense. Yet this presentation of overall intellectual ability, when verbal and nonverbal differences exist, continues to be performed by psychologists. As a result of

this gross culturally insensitive error, Alaska Natives have been unfairly labeled as intellectually disabled when, in fact, this is not the case.

2. To further validate and highlight an Alaska Native's relative strengths with nonverbal comprehension abilities, it is necessary to cross-validate the Wechsler intelligence scale with a sound nonverbal intelligence tool. The Leiter International Performance Scale, Leiter-3 (Stoelting Company, 2013), has filled this need for me. In my clinical experience, the Leiter-3 correlates strongly with the Wechsler Perceptual Reasoning index; when there are no statistically significant differences between the Wechsler verbal and nonverbal IQ indices, the Leiter-3 will correlate with the Full Scale IQ as well.

Cross-validating the Wechsler scale with the nonverbal Leiter gives me more confidence with the Wechsler results. And it provides me with more information to highlight the strengths of an Alaska Native, particularly when they demonstrate a relative weakness with verbal comprehension abilities compared to nonverbal comprehension skills.

I have also used the Comprehensive Test of Nonverbal Intelligence, CTONI-2 (PRO-ED, 2009). In my experience, however, the CTONI-2 does not consistently correlate with the Wechsler, and I have consequently stopped administering it to Alaska Natives in lieu of the Leiter-3. The only circumstance I have found the CTONI-2 correlating consistently with the Wechsler is when the individual is in the extremely low range of intellectual functioning.

In summary, the Wechsler Full Scale IQ cannot be used to provide an overall description of an Alaska Native's intellectual abilities when there are statistically significant differences between nonverbal and verbal comprehension composite scores. Interpreting the difference between verbal and nonverbal functioning is warranted. Further, cross-validating the Wechsler with the Leiter-3 potentially highlights the nonverbal strengths of Alaska Natives and gives more confidence to the examiner when reporting the Wechsler results. Although there are other nonverbal tests of intelligence, I have found the Leiter-3 superior with regard to correlating well with the Wechsler scale.

Emotional and Behavioral Functioning

Used worldwide, the Achenbach System of Empirically Based Assessment (ASEBA) has been useful with Alaska Natives, providing reliable measures of competencies, adaptive functioning, substance abuse, personal strengths, and behavioral, emotional, and social problems for clients of all ages. For youth, I habitually obtain assessments from parents and schoolteachers to evaluate and monitor behavior over time regarding home and school settings. For older individuals, such as adults undergoing assessment for dementia, I prefer to have adults who know the Elder well complete the Older Adult Behavior Checklist (OABCL).

The ASEBA tools can be augmented by other assessment instruments. For example, although the Attention Problems scale has been found accurate for screening for ADHD (see, for example, Raiker et al. 2017), I like to use the Conners 3, Parent and Teacher Short forms (Multi-Health Systems, Inc. 2008), to further capture ADHD symptoms within the home and school settings. Adding a computer-administered continuous performance test is also important when assessing for ADHD. The Test of Variables of Attention (TOVA) has filled this need for me.

Personality Functioning

Assessing personality functioning with Alaska Natives is not typically done. If it is a normal practice, I would question why this is happening, particularly in a rural setting. In my experience, a personality assessment is often done in the context of a legal situation where attorneys want a full formal psychological evaluation that includes personality assessment. Sometimes, too, medical providers would like a patient to undergo personality testing due to questions related to the individual's psychological functioning in light of their physical functioning.

Although I have used the Minnesota Multiphasic Personality Inventory—2nd Edition, MMPI-2 (Pearson), as well as the Millon Clinical Multiaxial Inventory, I have a much higher regard for the Personality Assessment Inventory (PAI; see www.parinc.com). The former two tests have fallen out of favor with me. The Millon, for example, was normed on a clinical population concentrating "on the differences in the diagnosis of clients, in comparison to other tests of mental health" (Lightfoot 2017, 1397); as such, it presents a potential bias if a mental health provider administers it to an Alaska Native client in a typical outpatient setting. I have found that the MMPI-2 frequently pathologizes Alaska Natives, which I attribute to its lack of sensitivity to the cultural nuances of my Alaska Native clients. For example, my Alaska Native clients often share spiritual experiences that, if taken out of their cultural context, present as psychotic phenomena. Desai's dissertation (2015), focused on using the MMPI-2 with Minnesota Native Americans, found elevations of the clinical scale 8 (Sc), which were attributed to the spiritual beliefs (e.g., having visions) shared in the Native American culture. In another study involving MMPI-2 with American Indians, Hill and her colleagues (2010) provide an astute critique: "From an Indigenous perspective, the MMPI-2 explicitly represents Western power and domination as an instrument that denies Indigenous people the right to psychological self-determination." They add: "the MMPI-2 is not an instrument that legitimates or even acknowledges Indigenous knowledges, worldviews, and experiences, but rather an instrument that legitimates and privileges hegemonic Western standards, norms, values, epistemology, and ontology" (24). In another study, Kagan's dissertation (2014) found higher MMPI-2 scores among American Indians compared to White participants, correlating with lesser degrees of acculturation with Native individuals.

To date I have found no studies exploring the use of the PAI among Alaska Natives. In my experience, however, the PAI provides a more grounded personality assessment that does not unfairly pathologize Alaska Natives. Obviously, more research is needed. Further, whenever I employ personality testing with Alaska Natives, I must have a sound referral question to support doing such testing. There must be some potential benefit to Alaska Natives undergoing personality assessments, or such evaluations should not be considered. This is true for general psychological evaluations as well. Indiscriminately performing psychological testing and/or personality assessments has the potential to unfairly pathologize Alaska Natives.

Other Tests I Have Used with Alaska Natives

- The Adaptive Behavior Assessment System, Third Edition, ABAS-3 (Western Psychological Services, 2015), providing an assessment of adaptive skills from birth to eighty-nine years
- The Delis-Kaplan Executive Function System, D-KEFS (The Psychological Corporation) for the assessment of verbal and non-verbal executive functions
- The NEPSY-II (Pearson) for the assessment of executive and memory functioning in preschool and school-age children
- The Wechsler Memory Scale—Fourth Edition, WMS-IV (Pearson) for memory and working memory abilities in individuals ages sixteen to ninety.
- The Repeatable Battery for the Assessment of Neuropsychological Status, RBANS (The Psychological Corporation)
- The Peabody Vocabulary Test (receptive) and the Expressive Vocabulary Test (Pearson)
- The Boehm Test of Basic Concepts (The Psychological Corporation), which provides a nice assessment of basic relational concepts important for language and cognitive development and later success in school for children ages three to five; it also

gives parents individual guidelines specific for teaching their children concepts they have not yet mastered.

Psychiatric Disorders, ACEs, Epigenetics, and Alaska Natives

High rates of adverse childhood experiences (ACEs) have been found among Native Americans (see, for example, Brockie, Heinzelmann, and Gill 2013; Brockie et al. 2015). This is true in my own clinical experience with Alaska Natives. Health disparities among Native Americans/Alaska Natives compared to other Americans also exist. Data gathered in a national study from 2001 to 2002 from the National Epidemiologic Survey on Alcohol and Related Conditions (Grant 2016) demonstrated a pattern of higher prevalence of psychiatric disorders among American Indians/Alaska Natives compared to non-Hispanic Whites. Current research links ACEs to risks related to health and well-being among American Indians and Alaska Natives. Yet the mechanisms underlying these risks are not clearly understood.

Although epigenetics research is in its infancy, epigenetics has been implicated in the understanding and the novel treatment of psychiatric disorders (Stahl 2009, 2010). The methylenetetrahydrofolate reductase (MTHFR) gene, for example, has been identified as pivotal in the metabolism of folate to methylated folate. It is estimated that about 40 percent of the general population has a deficiency on one half of the gene (heterozygous) and 20 percent of the population has a deficiency of the entire gene (homozygous). Deficiencies of the MTHFR gene limit the production of precursor amino acids necessary for the formation of serotonin, dopamine, and norepinephrine—contributing to emotional problems such as anxiety and depression (Hunt 2017). Further, individuals who have suffered from significant environmental stress such as childhood trauma have been linked to MTHFR polymorphisms (Lok et al. 2013).

In a randomized, double-blind, placebo-controlled study, Mech and Farah (2016) treated patients diagnosed with major depressive disorder and MTHFR polymorphism with reduced (metabolized) B vitamins and micronutrients, resulting in significant improvement in their symptoms compared to placebo patients; these results supported the therapeutic benefit of reduced B vitamins in the treatment of major depressive disorder, particularly with patients positive for MTHFR gene deficiencies.

Brockie (2013) and her colleagues articulate a framework incorporating ACEs, epigenetics, and high health disparities among Native Americans. She maintains that there is a mediating relationship of epigenetics contributing to health disparities among Native Americans with adverse childhood experiences. She provides evidence that psychiatric disorders are associated with methylation differences in genes that regulate the stress response, in addition to differences in endocrine, immune, and neurotransmitter genes that govern the stress response, although more research is needed to understand how ACEs contribute to health and well-being to better inform future interventions.

In the near future, as research already is demonstrating, our understanding of the MTHFR gene may make mental health work easier. Psychiatric nurse Russel Hunt (2017), for example, employs MTHR testing with his clients; further, he incorporates methylated folate as part of treatment, when indicated. Additionally, he asserts that relaxation and mental health well-being can be enhanced when clients accept and enforce these three rules: 1) no yelling; 2) no swearing; and 3) no name calling. When these three rules are practiced, people are more inclined to employ their frontal lobe in lieu of their limbic system. He habitually teaches these three rules to his clients who have shown compromised folate metabolism.

Clients who have suffered from childhood traumas and whose lives are subsequently filled with anxiety and depression can benefit from sober self-regulatory methods to calm themselves. It appears paramount that—regardless whether a mental health provider incorporates genetic testing with clients and methylated folate treatment—clients learn self-regulatory methods in lieu of alcohol and drug abuse for mitigating the sympathetic nervous system response when triggered. Appreciation of epigenetics reinforces this thesis.

Working with "Resistance" and Stages of Change, Community Readiness, and Healing

I have learned over the years that my response to "treatment-resistant clients" is a vital determinant to my becoming susceptible to emotional burnout. (For me, "treatment-resistant clients" are those clients who appear slow to make treatment progress for whatever reason.) Similar to my ocean experience, if I confront resistance head-on I am prone to making things worse for myself—and likely for my clients as well. And if I am not aware of what I am doing, my course can become more reckless through behaviors that are not conducive to creating a positive flow in my work. Further, I can set in motion internal cognitive activity that is not helpful to my health. As I experienced on the ocean, when I confronted the wind and the waves directly I was stymied and my canoe became perilously unstable. My thoughts, too, became irrational ("I need to make it to the island against this wind and current"), and such thinking set me off balance toward panic and despair.

I make a concerted attempt to consistently "move" with my clients and to accept them as they are. This is similar to motivational interviewing's principle of "roll with resistance" (Miller and Rollnick 2002). Instead of a physical entity like the wind and the waves, I am negotiating a perception. And there are many ways to work with a perception. But some main points, like those from Miller and Rollnick (2002), that I always try to keep in mind are:

- Avoid arguing for change.
- Resistance is not directly opposed.

- New perspectives are invited but not imposed.
- The client is a primary resource in finding answers and solutions.
- Resistance is a signal to respond differently (p. 40).

DiClemente and Velasquez's stages of change (2002) are useful for understanding the process of behavior change my clients go through, whether it is to initiate a new behavior, modify it, or terminate it altogether. In the treatment of substance use disorders, the newly revised resource from the Substance Abuse and Mental Health Services Administration *Enhancing Motivation for Change in Substance Use Disorder Treatment* (2019) provides specific motivational strategies for therapists for each stage of change. When I am mindful of these stages and the therapeutic strategies suited to them, I find myself more at ease with the process, the journey that I am on with my "treatment-resistant clients," particularly those struggling with substance use. And I am more apt to accept my clients as they are and to recognize and appreciate the successful actions they are engaging in. Being in tune with the stages of change helps me reaffirm the decisions my clients make and, in this manner, keeps me on a path that reinforces and is aligned with self-determination and the strengths perspective. I become a partner in my client's change process.

Similar to emotional burnout when working with "resistant" clients, I sometimes find myself prone to burnout when I perceive a community (Native or non-Native) seemingly failing to address issues such as alcoholism. Like the personal stages of change, the community readiness model (CRM) developed by the Tri-Ethnic Center for Prevention Research (Plested, Jumper-Thurman, and Edwards 2016) helps me maintain a developmental framework that appreciates the process of community development. It provides a broad medium for understanding the degree to which a community is willing and prepared to take action on an issue. Like the personal stages of change, CRM helps me accept a community as it is without judgment. And it helps me understand the internal change processes necessary to move communities forward toward addressing an issue.

Further punctuating the equation of the community readiness model is the concept of community healing developed by Lane (2002) and his colleagues with Four Directions International and the Four Worlds Centre for Development Learning. It grew from a need to articulate the strategies that promote healing within Aboriginal Canadian communities. The four phases of community healing include:

1. The Journey Begins: A core group of people begin to address their own healing needs. People feel safe enough to share their personal stories of pain and dysfunction.
2. Gathering Momentum: Healing activities are increased, coupled with people looking at the root causes of addiction, abuse, and violence through community-wide awareness workshops.
3. Hitting the Wall: Building healing capacity continues, but many frontline workers feel burned out since the process appears to have stalled. There is a growing awareness that not only individuals need to heal but whole systems as well. The honeymoon stage is over, and the difficult work of changing entrenched community patterns, steeped in oppression and dysfunction, has begun. A new community identity is commencing.
4. From Healing to Transformation: A significant change in community consciousness is taking place—shifting from fixing problems to transforming systems. (59–72)

When I consider the community readiness model and the phases of community healing, I am reminded of the video *The Honour of All, the Story of Alkali Lake* (Four Worlds International Institute for Human and Community Development 2006). It eloquently illustrates how the dynamics of cultural and spiritual destruction between 1940 and 1985 impacted the Shuswap people and led to local, grassroots efforts to restore healing to their culture and sobriety from alcohol to their community. I habitually show this DVD to my clients to reinforce their own efforts in recovery from alcohol on an individual and community level.

Self-Care

At a funeral for an individual who committed suicide, I was approached by a community leader who bluntly said, "If this continues, we're going to cut the counseling program because it is not working." It was a moot point, at that moment, to mention to the community leader that the person who committed suicide had never sought out mental health services with me or any other village-based mental health provider. Still, his words cut deeply into my sense of self as a mental health provider.

Working in a rural region and being the major mental health resource can place responsibility on us whether it is deserved or not. As one Native colleague said, "We are blamed sometimes for all the bad things that happen." Working in a small community, compared to a city where resources are readily available and where resources can also absorb the responsibility whether it is deserved or not, makes the emotional toll on mental health providers quite poignant. After serving my first seven years in the Bering Strait region, I left the profession altogether for fifteen months to recover from burnout.

I am not proud to state that I have dealt with the suicidal deaths of several Native clients. One might say that this is statistically inevitable, given my working over two decades in an area of Alaska known for its highest suicide rate, at more than six times the national average and four times than the state average. Still, I often look back at those who died and wonder if I could have done anything differently.

To prevent emotional burnout, I strive to practice balance. Having a family, for instance, compared to when I was single in my earlier years, has forced me to budget my time between work and family, although I am still prone to working overtime. I am also acutely mindful of the interaction between my feelings, thoughts, and behavior (see Figure 1). For example, when I am tired at the end of a workday, I may feel depressed. To combat these depressive symptoms I immerse myself in the aerobic behavior of jogging either on a treadmill or outside when the weather is favorable. I am consistently amazed how exercise such as running lifts me from my depressive mindset. I feel balanced after becoming physically tired. Once grounded, I am able to engage in more rational, healthy thinking. This is, of course, what works for me, and it may not work for others. But it underscores the importance for mental health providers to find what best promotes balance in their life.

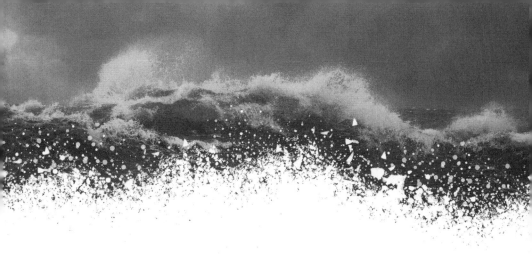

CHAPTER SIX

Prevention Considerations

A s previously emphasized (see Droby 2000), when working within Alaska Native communities, mental health providers must be mindful of the paradigm of prevention: primary prevention services (e.g., suicide prevention education) designed to prevent problems from ever occurring within a population; secondary prevention services targeted at groups at risk for developing a problem (e.g., encouraging stress-reducing strategies for people prone to anxiety); and tertiary prevention services focused on reducing the impact of an existing problem (e.g., support groups for people dealing with loss). Having a crisis-oriented mindset can make us lose track of the bigger picture of mitigating risks for problem behaviors. Further, it can make us less aware of the positive protective factors existing within a Native community. By recognizing the paradigm of prevention, mental health providers have more avenues to negotiate in the current of activities within a Native community. Romano (2015) reminds us that enhancing personal and social

Guiding Principles

Self-determination is possible for Alaska Natives

Native self-determination is best promoted through decentralized mental health services

The role of the non-Native mental health professional imparts a co-participatory and background presence

The role of the non-Native mental health professional is multifaceted and collectively mindful

Cultural Considerations $\updownarrow$

Mindset, transference, and the strengths of Alaska Native communities

Collective colonizing trauma and specific traumas on Native communities

Culture of silence

Collectivism

Therapy Considerations $\updownarrow$

Relational-cultural theory

Relational-cultural therapy (RCT) and multicultural care

Psychotherapy with Alaska Natives

Initial treatment engagement

Parenting and the use of parent-child interaction therapy (PCIT)

Strengths perspective

Trauma-focused narrative therapy with children

Crisis intervention

Psychotropic medication

Bibliotherapy

Adjunctive Considerations

Self-determination versus dependency

Dependency patterns

Colonization patterns

Tribal problems, tribal solutions

 Personal biases/worldview

Generalist orientation

Hurting helpers

Personal well-being (PWB)

Native spirituality

Native identity

The assets study

Flow

Tribal healers

Learning and communication styles

 Maslow's Hierarchy Of Needs

Trust/mistrust

Working with schools in Alaska Native communities

Ethics

Psychological testing and Alaska Natives

Psychiatric disorders, ACEs, epigenetics and Alaska Natives

 Working with resistance and stages of change, community readiness and healing

Self-care

Prevention Considerations $\updownarrow$

Primary

$\leftrightarrow$ Secondary

Tertiary

Figure 4. The dynamic flow of multifaceted factors for mental health practices in Alaska Native communities.

well-being in the field of prevention psychology involves the "need to consider both risk and protection variables" (63).

Figure 4 illustrates the elements of my model, underscored by the prevention paradigm. These elements are not static but are often interrelated and move fluidly like the wind and the waves.

I have been honored through the years to have worked alongside BHAs and BHPs in Native communities in a multitude of prevention activities: subsistence activities with youth at fish camps led by Elders, teaching PCIT to Head Start teachers and parents, role modeling self-regulatory methods for dealing with stress in prosocial ways in school classrooms, participating in puppet demonstrations of alcohol-related family problems to kindergarteners, participating in community talking circles so late into the night that the next day the schoolteachers complained of their students sleeping in class, solution-building workshops addressing problems within the community, presenting the dynamics of suicide and role modeling ways for community members to connect with people who are in crisis and contemplating self-harm, serving on local advisory boards addressing CRM and village action plans, teaching assets to parents, and winter camping with youth.

Prevention psychology substantially widens the field of mental health work within a Native community, particularly for BHAs and BHPs. Further, I have observed that those BHAs/BHPs who strongly embrace prevention within their communities have a high degree of credibility and respect. Hopefully, in the near future BHAs/BHPs will be able to bill for prevention activities since such services are critical to rural behavioral health in Alaska and also core to the BHA scope of practice (Alaska Native Tribal Health Consortium, personal communication, 2017).

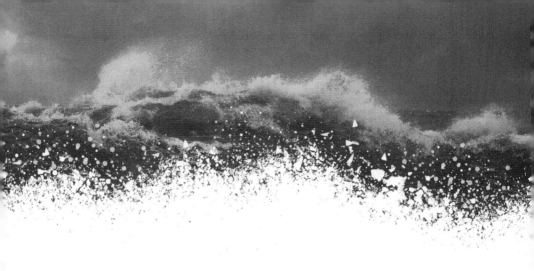

CHAPTER SEVEN

Concluding Thoughts

Working as a mental health provider in a Native village, I sometimes find myself paddling with all my strength against a difficult current, meeting only frustration, fatigue, doubt, and a sense of helplessness. During these times, my sense of self becomes precariously unstable. Sometimes I find myself negotiating heavy water where my perceived progress is slow and laborious, as if I am paddling with no apparent positive movement. I remind myself during these times not to become paralyzed. Rather, I am inspired by the words of Duran (2006) to embrace humility in my work and to not become undone in the difficult healing process of my Native clients. I am reminded, too, of the words of LaDue (1994), who advises non-Native mental health professionals to closely examine their motives for working with Native people, since Native people "do not need any more people who want to 'do something' for us, 'rescue our poor children,' 'save our souls'" (106). And I remind myself to change course in the throes of my frustration and to move with the current and recapture the strength that is offered by the wind and the waves, the strengths that exist within Native communities if only I open my eyes and widen my field of awareness. I become mindful of how pushing against the current only serves to make things worse. I change course and roll with the pain and the hurt that is not a Native phenomenon but rather a human phenomenon, one that is more readily observed and felt in a small community such as a Native village in Alaska.

Further, I take stock of the stages of change my clients are in to appreciate the process of human development. I pause, too, to remember the clients I have worked with who have successfully negotiated problems in their lives. I am reminded of the dynamics that appear central to all these treatment cases: (1) problems (e.g., trauma, stressors) are managed without the use of substances; (2) clients have a strong sober support system, particularly with their significant others, who also demonstrate no problems with substance abuse; and (3) clients consistently have a life filled with purpose, often highly connected to their culture, their families, and communities, and possess a strong desire to be a positive role model to their children, to themselves, and to the youth in their villages. This latter point underscores successful clients having an integral connection with people rather than with alcohol and/or other drugs.

Having a relationship with drugs rather than people is a significant distraction to successful treatment. To illustrate this relational point, I am reminded of a woman who became sober from her addiction to smoking cannabis. She once shared with me that in the depths of her addiction she would lie on her living room floor, immersed in the haze of cannabis, while her one- and two-year-old children played in the middle of a heavily traveled street in her village. She explained: "When I was addicted to pot, I would just lay there, knowing my children were unsupervised, and I could care less. Smoking pot was the only thing that mattered to me." Now that she was sober, this woman was consistently amazed at how her relationship with cannabis had taken the place of her relationship with family. She would never again entertain placing her children secondary to her use of cannabis.

When I am riding the wind and the waves, I am reminded that I have been privileged to observe firsthand the resiliency of the human spirit. How, in spite of personal struggles, there still is hope to heal from wounds in the past and wounds currently experienced. I witness people embracing sober living and dealing with their feelings without medicating them. I observe people recapturing memories from their past and living with them in a more manageable manner. I observe people reclaiming their culture—dancing into the night and subsisting during the day, picking berries, smoking fish, beading, sewing, teaching their children their Native language, and sharing with each other in the spirit of authentic generosity. And I observe that there is hope to break the cycle of hurt that has been passed on from generation to generation, from childhood to parenthood, for many Native people.

As a non-Native mental health provider, I do not posture as a "wannebe-Native," or as a Native healer who does prayer smoke with his Native clients or engages them in a traditional Native dance to invoke a sense of cultural identity, spirituality and healing. I am comfortable with who I am, aware of my shortcomings and strengths. I have no need to impose my beliefs on people and make them into a person like myself. I am a good listener, empathic and attentive to the strengths of my clients. I provide a safe, confidential space for them to share their problems and concerns. And I am comfortable with implementing some method of trauma-informed psychotherapy should my clients choose to go there. I exercise mindfulness, too, toward the historical context my Native clients have lived and experienced generationally. And I enhance awareness of the "soul wound" or trauma they have suffered and collaboratively explore avenues to heighten mental health wellness and develop prosocial coping strategies to deal with stress. Further, I also extend mindfulness toward myself and my own history of trauma so that I do not unfairly transfer unresolved issues to my Native clients.

I am aware of my limitations and accept the uncertainty of performing mental health work: I know I cannot predict the choices my clients exercise in their lives, and I learn ways to personally cope in a healthy manner with the unfortunate consequences that sometimes occur with people struggling with an inordinate amount of stressors. Within this web of working, I am sensitive to the therapeutic relationship and consistently cultivate a supportive, healing bond of interaction. And I am cognizant of the colonizing legacy that has impacted Native individuals, their families, and their communities. I make a concerted effort to ensure my presence does not add to this harmful history. I consider myself a guest when I am in Native country, on Native land, and I am consistently critiquing how I behave as a guest.

Some people may argue that the therapeutic elements and model I have articulated here—addressing accumulated hurt, grief, and learned responses to trauma—ignores larger factors embedded at the societal level in politics and economics. Assimilationist policies that have undermined Alaska Native people and their land, subsistence, and their power toward self-government have long been recognized (Berger, 1985; Hensley, 2009). Indeed, there are many dimensions, many influences impacting Alaska Natives. As a mental health provider in a Native community I recognize these elements and am not naive and dismissive to them. At the same time, I do not let these larger factors distract me from doing my job, from working and connecting with individuals who are hurting and sitting before me in my office or in their home or in a village jail.

I remember the words of Margaret Mead: "Never doubt that a small group of thoughtful, committed citizens can change the world; indeed, it's the only thing that ever has." I recall the Shuswap community, led by the Chelsea family of Alkali Lake, British Columbia, and the journey of healing they undertook toward embracing sobriety from a village steeped in alcoholism. And I am reminded of the words I once read on the wall of a café while traveling in Viet Nam: "To the world you may be one person. But to one person you may be the world."

It has not been easy for the people of village Alaska to be heard.
For many years, they have been caught up in the
cultural uncertainties of assimilationist policies.

—*Thomas R. Berger (1985)*

We will be heard, in the wind, on the water,
and in the quiet dignity of our old ones:
The people speak: Will YOU listen?

—*Robin A. LaDue (1994)*

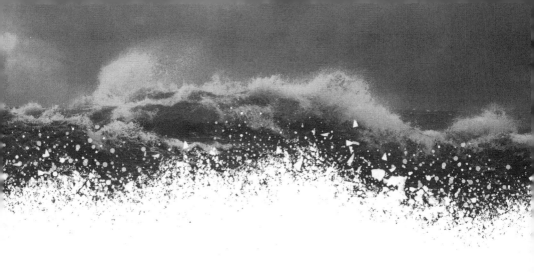

References

Alaska Native Tribal Health Consortium. (2014). *Doorway to a Sacred Place*. State of Alaska, Alaska Department of Health and Social Services, Division of Behavioral Health.

Allen, J. (2002). Assessment Training for Practice in American Indian and Alaska Native Settings. *Journal of Personality Assessment*, 79 (2), 216–225.

Allen, J., Mohatt, G., Fok, C., Henry, D. and Burkett, R. (2014). A Protective Factors Model for Alcohol Abuse and Suicide Prevention Among Alaska Native Youth. *American Journal of Community Psychology*, 54 (0), 125–139.

Allen, J., Mohatt, G., Beehler, S. and Rowe, H. (2014). People Awakening: Collaborative Research to Develop Cultural Strategies for Prevention in Community Intervention. *American Journal of Community Psychology*, 54 (0), 100–111.

Allen, J. and Mohatt, G. (2014). Introduction to Ecological Description of a Community Intervention: Building Prevention through Collaborative Field Based Research. *American Journal of Community Psychology*, 54 (0), 83–90.

Aronson, E., Wilson, T. D. and Akert, R. M. (2013). *Social Psychology*. Upper Saddle River, NJ: Pearson Education, Inc.

Association of Alaska School Boards. (1998). *Helping Kids Succeed—Alaskan Style*. Juneau, AK: Department of Health and Human Services.

Association of Alaska School Boards' Alaska Initiative for Community Engagement. (2003). *Helping Little Kids Succeed—Alaskan Style*. Juneau, AK: Department of Health and Human Services.

Atkinson, D. R. (2004). *Counseling American Minorities*. New York: The McGraw-Hill Companies, Inc.

Atkinson, M. (2010). *Resurrection After Rape*. Oklahoma City, OK: Rar Publishing.

Bachelor, A. (1988). How Clients Perceive Therapist Empathy: A Content Analysis of Received Empathy. *Psychotherapy*, 25, 227–240.

Baranowsky, A. B. and Gentry, J. E. (2015). *Trauma Practice*. Boston, MA: Hogrefe Publishing.

Baschnagel, J. S., Coffey, S. F. and Rash, C. J. (2006). The Treatment of Co-Occurring PTSD and Substance Use Disorders Using Trauma-Focused Exposure Therapy. *International Journal of Behavioral Consultation and Therapy*, 2 (4), 498–508.

Bates, T. (2015). The Glass Is Half Full and Half Empty: A Population-Representative Twin Study Testing If Optimism and Pessimism Are Distinct Systems. *The Journal of Positive Psychology*, 1–9.

Benson, P. L., Galbraith, J. and Espeland, P. (1995). *What Kids Need to Succeed*. Minneapolis, MN: Free Spirit Publishing Inc.

Berg, I. (1994). *Family-Based Services: A Solution-Focused Approach*. New York: W. W. Norton and Company.

Berg, I. and De Shazer, S. (1994). *A Tap on the Shoulder*. Audiotape by the Brief Family Therapy Center, Milwaukee, WI.

Berg, I. and Reuss, N. (1998). *Solutions Step by Step*. New York: W. W. Norton and Company.

Berger, T. (1985). *Village Journey*. New York: Hill and Wang.

Bergquist, P. (2010). *The Long Dark Winter's Night: Reflections of a Priest in a Time of Pain and Privilege*. Collegeville, MN: Order of Saint Benedict.

Berry, J. W. (1990). Psychology of Acculturation: Understanding Individuals Moving Between Cultures. *Applied Cross-Cultural Psychology*, 232–253.

Berry, J. W. (1997). Immigration, Acculturation, and Adaptation. *Applied Psychology: An International Review*, 46 (1), 5–68.

Berry, J. W. (2005). Acculturation: Living Successfully in Two Cultures. *International Journal of Intercultural Relations*, 29, 697–712.

Berry, J. W., Kim, U., Power, S., Young, M. and Bajaki, M. (1989). Acculturation Attitudes in Plural Societies. *Applied Psychology: An International Review, 38* (2), 185–206.

Berry, J. W., Trimble, J. E. and Olmedo, E. L. (1986). Assessment of Acculturation. In: Berry, J. W. and Lonner, W. J. (Eds.), *Field Methods in Cross Cultural Research*. Thousand Oaks, CA: Sage.

Bigfoot, D. S. (2011). The Process and Dissemination of Cultural Adaptations of Evidence-Based Practices for American Indian and Alaska Native Children and Their Families. In Sarche, M. C., Spicer, P., Farrell, P. and Fitzgerald, H. E. (Eds.), *American Indian and Alaska Native Children and Mental Health* (Pp. 285–307). Santa Barbara, CA: Praeger.

Bigfoot, D. S. and Funderburk, B. W. (2011). Honoring Children, Making Relatives: The Cultural Translation of Parent-Child Interaction Therapy for American Indian and Alaska Native Families. *Journal of Psychoactive Drugs, 43* (4), 309–318.

Bigfoot, D. S. and Schmidt, S. R. (2010). Honoring Children, Mending the Circle: Cultural Adaptation of Trauma-Focused Cognitive-Behavioral Therapy for American Indian and Alaska Native Children. *Journal of Clinical Psychology 66* (8), 847–856.

Bopp, M. & Bopp, J. (2006). *Re-creating the world*. Alberta, Canada: Four Worlds Press.

Brave Heart, M. Y. H., Lewis-Fernandez, R., Beals, J., Hasin, D. S., Sugaya, L., Wang, S., Grant, B. G. and Blanco, C. (2016). Psychiatric Disorders and Mental Health Treatment in American Indians and Alaska Natives: Results of the National Epidemiologic Survey on Alcohol and Related Conditions. *Social Psychiatry Psychiatric Epidemiology, 51*, 1033–1046.

Breslau, N., Davis, G. C. and Schultz, L. R. (2003). Posttraumatic Stress Disorder and the Incidence of Nicotine, Alcohol, and Other Drug Disorders in Persons Who Have Experienced Trauma. *Archives of General Psychiatry, 60*, 289–294.

Brockie, T. N., Heinzelmann, M. and Gill, J. (2013). A Framework to Examine the Role of Epigenetics in Health Disparities Among Native Americans. *Nursing Research and Practice, 2013*.

Brockie, T. N., Dana-Sacco, G., Wallen, G. R., Wilcox, H. C. and Campbell, J. C. (2015). The Relationship of Adverse Childhood Experiences to PTSD, Depression, Poly-Drug Use and Suicide Attempt in Reservation-Based Native American Adolescents and Young Adults. *American Journal of Community Psychology, 55*, 411–421.

Burdick, D. (2016). *ADHD: Non-Medication Treatments and Skills for Children and Teens*. Eau Claire, WI: Pesi Publishing and Media.

Burdick, D. (2013). *Mindfulness Skills Workbook: For Clinicians and Clients*. Eau Claire, WI: Pesi Publishing and Media.

Butler, M., Carroll, K., Roeser, P., Soza War Soldier, R., Walker, S., Woodruff, L. (2005). Decolonizing Methodologies: Research and Indigenous Peoples, and: Peace, Power and Righteousness: An Indigenous Manifesto (Review). *The American-Indian Quarterly*, 29 (1 and 2), 288–292.

Carroll, J. (2019). To Save the Church, Dismantle the Priesthood. *The Atlantic*, June.

Chatzky, J. (2003). *You Don't Have to Be Rich*. New York: Penguin Group.

Clayton, Manning, Krygsman and Speiser. (2017). *Mental Health and Our Changing Climate: Impacts, Implications, and Guidance*. Washington, D.C.: American Psychological Association, and Ecoamerica.

Comas-Diaz, L. (2012). *Multicultural Care: A Clinician's Guide to Cultural Competence*. Washington, D.C.: American Psychological Association.

Conner, T., Deyoung, C. and Silvia, P. (2016). Everyday Creative Activity As a Path to Flourishing. *The Journal of Positive Psychology*, 1–9.

Craig, G. (2011). *The eft manual*. Santa Rosa, CA: Energy Psychology Press.

Csikszentmihalyi, M. (1990). *Flow*. New York: HarperCollins Publishers.

Danese, Moffitt, Harrington, Milne, Polanczyk, Pariante, Poulton and Caspi. (2009). *Adverse childhood experiences and adult risk factors for age-related disease*. Archives of Pediatric Adolescent Medicine, 163 (12), 1135–1143.

David, E. J. R. (2014). *Internalized Oppression*. New York: Springer Publishing Company, LLC.

Day, Provost and Lanier. (2006). *Alaska native mortality update: 1999–2003*. Anchorage, AK; Alaska Native Epidemiology Center, Office of Alaska Native Health Research, Division of Community Health Services, Alaska Native Tribal Health Consortium.

Decou, C. R., Skewes, M. C. and Lopez, E. (2013). Traditional Living and Cultural Ways As Protective Factors Against Suicide: Perceptions of Alaska Native University Students. *International Journal of Circumpolar Health*, 72 1–10.

De Graff, J., Wann, D. and Naylor, T. H. (2005). *Affluenza: The All-Consuming Epidemic*. San Francisco, CA: Berrett-Koehler Publishers, Inc.

Dejong, P. and Berg, K. (1998). *Interviewing for Solutions*. Pacific Grove, CA: Brooks/Cole.

Desai, K. (2015). *Clinician perspectives on culturally sensitive mmpi-2 interpretation*. Minneapolis, MN: A Clinical Dissertation Submitted to the Graduate Faculty of Saint Mary's University of Minnesota in Partial Fullfillment of the Requirements for the Degree of Doctor of Psychology in Counseling Psychology. Ann Arbor, MI: ProQuest LLC (#3739829).

DiClemente, C. C. and Velasquez, M. M. (2002). Motivational Interviewing and the Stages of Change. In *Motivational Interviewing* (Pp. 201–216). New York: The Guilford Press.

Dodge Rea, B. (2001). Finding Our Balance: The Investigation and Clinical Application of Intuition. *Psychotherapy, 38,* 97–106.

Doyle, T. P., Sipe, A. W. and Wall, P. J. (2006). *Sex, Priests, and Secret Codes: The Catholic Church's 2000-Year Paper Trail of Sexual Abuse.* Los Angeles, CA: Volt Press.

Droby, R. (2000). *With the Wind and the Waves.* Norton Sound Health Corporation.

Duncan, B. L., Hubble, M. A. and Miller, S. D. (1997). *Psychotherapy with "Impossible" Cases.* New York: W. W. Norton and Company, Inc.

Duran, E. (2006). *Healing the Soul Wound.* New York: Teachers College Press.

Duran, E. and B. Duran. (1995). *Native American Postcolonial Psychology.* Albany, NY: State University of New York.

Eisenberger, N. I. (2012). The Neural Bases of Social Pain: Evidence for Shared Representations with Physical Pain. *Psychosomatic Medicine, 74* (2), 126–135.

Eisenberger, N. I., Lieberman, M. D. and Williams, K. D. (2003). Does Rejection Hurt? An FMRI Study of Social Exlusion. *Science, 302,* 290–292.

Federal Register. (December 2014). *United States Department of Justice Attorney General Guidelines Stating Principles for Working with Federally Recognized Indian Tribes.* Washington, D.C.: Office of the Attorney General.

Feinstein, D. (2018). Energy Psychology: Efficacy, Speed, Mechanisms. *Explore,* 1–15.

Felitti, V. J., Anda, R. F., Nordenberg, D., Williamson, D. F., Spitz, A. M., Edwards, V., Koss, M. P. and Marks, J. S. (1998). Relationship of Childhood Abuse and Household Dysfunction to Many of the Leading Causes of Death in Adults. *American Journal of Preventive Medicine, 14,* 245–258.

Feuereison, P. (2005). *Invisible Girls.* Emeryville, CA: Seal Press.

Fienup-Riordan, A. *Eskimo essays: Yup'ik lives and how we see them.* New Brunswick, N.J., & London: Rutgers University Press.

Flint, G. A., Lammers, W. and Mitnick, D. G. (2006). Emotional Freedom Techniques: A Safe Treatment Intervention for Many Trauma Based Issues. *Journal of Aggression, Maltreatment and Trauma, 12* (1), 125–150.

Foa, E. B., Zoellner, L. A., Feeny, N. C., Hembree, E. A. and Alvarez-Conrad, J. (2002). Does Imaginal Exposure Exacerbate PTSD Symptoms? *Journal of Consulting and Clinical Psychology, 70* (4), 1022–1028.

Fok, C. C. T., Allen, J. and Henry, D. (2014). The Brief Family Relationship Scale: A Brief Measure of the Relationship Dimension in Family Functioning. *Assessment, 21* (1), 67–72.

Foulks, E. F. (1989). Misalliances in the Barrow Alcohol Study. *American Indian and Native Alaska Mental Health Research, 2* (3), 7–17.

Four Worlds International Institute for Human and Community Development. (2006). DVD: *The Honour of All, the Story of Alkali Lake*. Surrey, British Columbia: Four Worlds International Institute for Human and Community Development.

Frankl, V. E. (1959). *Man's Search for Meaning*. Boston, MA: Beacon Press.

Freire, P. (1970). *Pedagogy of the Oppressed*. New York: The Continuum Publishing Corporation.

Freitas-Murrell, B. and Swift, J. K. (2015). Predicting Attitudes Toward Seeking Professional Help Among Alaska Natives. *American Indian and Alaska Native Mental Health Research, 22* (3), 21–35.

Frew, J. and Spiegler, M. (2008). Introduction to Contemporary Psychotherapies for a Diverse World. In J. Frew and M. Spiegler (Eds.), *Contemporary Psychotherapies for a Diverse World* (Pp. 1–9). New York: Lahaska Press.

Frontline. (2011). *The Silence*. Corporation for Public Broadcasting: ShopPBS. Org.

Gallagher, M., Lopez, S. and Pressman, S. (2013). Optimism Is Universal: Exploring the Presence and Benefits of Optimism in a Representative Sample of the World. *Journal of Personality, 81* (5), 429–440.

Gentry, J. E. (2014). Two-Day Trauma Digital Conference: Evidence-Based Trauma Treatments and Interventions and the 10 Core Competencies of Trauma, Ptsd, Grief and Loss. Eau Claire, WI: Pesi, Inc.

Gentry, J. E. (2016). *Forward Facing Trauma Therapy*. Sarasota, FL: Compassion Unlimited.

Giago, T. (2006). *Children Left Behind: The Dark Legacy of Indian Mission Boarding Schools*. Santa Fe, NM: Clear Light Publishing.

Gonzales, E. (2019). Meghan Markle and Prince Harry Are Launching a Show with Oprah for Apple. *Harper's Bazaar*, April 10.

Grandbois, D. (2005). Stigma of Mental Illness Among American Indian and Alaska Native Nations: Historical and Contemporary Perspectives. *Issues in Mental Health Nursing, 26*, 1001–1024.

Grant, B. (2016). *The National Epidemiologic Survey on Alcohol and Related Conditions*. Rockville, MD: U.S. Institutes of Health.

Hamilton, C. and Denniss, R. (2005). *Affluenza: When Too Much Is Never Enough*. Crows Nest, Nsw, Australia: Allen and Unwin.

Hartman, D. and Zimberoff, D. (2004). Corrective Emotional Experience in the Therapeutic Process. *Journal of Heart-Centered Therapies, 7* (2), 3–84.

Hawkins, P. and Shohet, R. (2012). *Supervision in the Helping Professions*. New York: Open University Press.

Hays, P. a. (2006). Cognitive-Behavioral Therapy with Alaska Native People. In: *Culturally Responsive Cognitive-Behavioral Therapy* (Ed. S)

Healthy Alaskans Partnership Council. (2010). *Healthy Alaskans, Volume II: Creating Healthy Communities*. Juneau, AK: Department of Health and Human Services.

Hembree, E. A., Foa, E. B., Dorfan, N. M., Street, G. P., Kowalski, J. and Tu, X. (2003). Do Patients Drop Out Prematurely from Exposure Therapy for PTSD? *Journal of Traumatic Stress, 16* (6), 555–562.

Hembree-Kigin, T. L. and McNeil, C. B. (1995) *Parent-Child Interaction Therapy*. New York: Plenum Press.

Hensely, W. (2009). *Fifty miles to tomorrow*. New York: Farrar, Straus and Giroux.

Herman, J. L. (1992). *Trauma and Recovery*. New York: Basic Books.

Hill, J. S., Pace, T. M. and Robbins, R. R. (2010). Decolonizing Personality Assessment and Honoring Indigenous Voices: A Critical Examination of the MMPI-2. *Cultural Diversity and Ethnic Minority Psychology, 16* (1), 16–25.

Hogan, M., Christopherson, S. and Rothe, A. (2006). *Formerly Used Defense Sites in the Norton Sound Region: Location, History of Use, Contaminants Present, and Status of Clean-Up Efforts*. National Institute of Environmental Health Sciences (NIEHS).

Holck, Day, and Provost. (2013). *Mortality trends among Alaska Native people: successes and challenges*, International Journal of Circumpolar Health, 72, 21185.

Hovey, D. (2019). Warmer Waters Investigated As Cause of Pink Salmon Die-off in Norton Sound Region. *Anchorage Daily News*, July 12.

Hunt, R. (2017, September 6). Workshop: *Using Genetics, Epigenetics and CBT to Treat Trauma, or Anything Else*. San Diego, CA.

Jacobsen, L. K., Southwick, S. M. and Kosten, T. R. (2001). Substance Use Disorders in Patients with Posttraumatic Stress Disorder: A Review of the Literature. *American Journal of Psychiatry*, *158* (8), 1184–1190.

Jayawickreme, E., Forgeard, M. and Seligman, M. (2012). The Engine of Well-Being. *Review of General Psychology*, *16*, 327–342.

Jordan, J. V. (2010). *Relational-Cultural Therapy*. Washington, D.C.: American Psychological Association.

Kagan, C. A. (2014). Impact of Cultural Identity on MMPI-2 Profiles in Northern Plains American Indians. Grand Forks, ND: A Dissertation Submitted to the Graduate Faculty of the University of North Dakota in Partial Fulfillment of the Requirements for the Degree Doctor of Philosophy.

Kaplan, L. and Girard, J. (1994). *Strengthening High-Risk Families: A Handbook for Practitioners*. New York: Wiley and Sons, Inc.

Kivimaki, M., Vahtera, J., Elovainio, M., Helenius, H., Singh-Manoux, A. and Pentti, J. (2005). Optimism and Pessimism As Predictors of Change in Health After Death or Onset of Severe Illness in Family. *Health Psychology*, *24* (4), 413–421.

Korn, L. (2017). *Eat Right, Feel Right: Over 80 Recipes and Tips to Improve Mood, Sleep, Attention and Focus*. Eau Claire, WI: Pesi, Inc.

Koss-Chioino, J. D. (2006). Spiritual Transformation, Relation, and Radical Empathy: Core Components of the Ritual Healing Process. *Transcultural Psychiatry*, *43*, 652–670.

Kral, R. and Kowalski, K. (1989). After the Miracle: The Second Stage in Solution Focused Brief Therapy. *Journal of Strategic and Systemic Therapies*, *8* (2–3), 73–76.

Lane, P., Bopp, M., Bopp, J. and Norris, J. (2002). *Mapping the Healing Journey: The Final Report of a National Research Project on Healing in Canadian Aboriginal Communities*. Ottawa, Canada: The Aboriginal Healing Foundation and Aboriginal Corrections Policy Unit.

LaDue, R. (1994). Coyote Returns: Twenty Sweats Does Not an Indian Expert Make. In N. Gartrell (Ed.). *Bringing Ethics Alive: Feminist Ethics in Psychotherapy Practice* (Pp. 93–111). New York: The Haworth Press, Inc.

Leung, C., Tsang, S., Sin, T. C. S. and Choi, S. (2015). The Efficacy of Parent-Child Interaction Therapy with Chinese Families: Randomized Controlled Trial. *Research on Social Work Practice*, *25* (1), 117–128.

Lewis, J. P. and Allen, J. (2017). Alaska Native Elders in Recovery: Linkages Between Indigenous Cultural Generativity and Sobriety to Promote Successful Aging. *Journal of Cross-Cultural Gerontology*, *28* (2).

Lightfoot, Jr., J. M. (2017). Critical Analysis of the Millon Clinical Multiaxial Inventory. *International Journal of Scientific and Engineering Research, 8* (1), 1397–1399.

Lok, A., Bockting, C. L. H., Koeter, M. W. J., Sneider, H., Mocking, R. J. T., Vinkers, Kahn, R. S., Boks, J. P. and Schene, A. H. (2013). Interaction Between the MTHFR C677t Polymorphism and Traumatic Childhood Events Predicts Depression. *Translational Psychiatry, 3.*

Lyubomirsky, S. and Layous, K. (2013). How Do Simple Positive Activities Increase Well-Being? *Association for Psychological Science,* 57–62.

Macdonald, J. P., Ford, J. D., Cunsolo, A. and Ross, N. (2013). A Review of Protective Factors and Causal Mechanisms That Enhance the Mental Health of Indigenous Circumpolar Youth. *International Journal of Circumpolar Health, 72,* 1–23.

Macdonald, J. P., Willox, A. C., Ford, J. D., Shiwak, I. and Wood, M. (2015). Protective Factors for Mental Health and Well-Being in a Changing Climate: Perspectives from Inuit Youth in Nunatsiavut, Labrador. *Social Science and Medicine, 141,* 133–141.

Marrs, J. (1997). *Alien Agenda.* New York: HarperCollins Publishers, Inc.

Masters, J. C., Burish, T. G., Hollon, S. D. and Rimm, D.C. (1987). *Behavior Therapy.* Orlando, FL: Harcourt Brace Jovanovich, Inc.

Mcnally, R. J., Bryant, R. A. and Ehlers, A. (2003). Does Early Psychological Intervention Promote Recovery from Posttraumatic Stress? *American Psychological Society, 4* (2), 45–79.

Mech, A. W. and Farah, A. (2016). Correlation of Clinical Response with Homocysteine Reduction During Therapy with Reduced B Vitamins in Patients with MDD Who Are Positive for MTHFR C677t or A1298c Polymorphism: A Randomized, Double-Blind, Placebo-Controlled Study. *Journal of Clinical Psychiatry, 77* (5), 668–671.

Mee-Lee, D., Mclellan, A. T. and Miller, S. D. (2010). What Works in Substance Abuse and Dependence Treatment. In: *The Heart and Soul of Change,* Duncan, B. L., Miller, S. D., Wampold, B. E. and Hubble, M. A. (Ed. S). Washington, D.C.: American Psychological Association, 393–417.

Mehl-Madrona, L. (2007). *Narrative Medicine.* Rochester, VT: Bear and Co.

Mele, C. and Victor, D. (2016). Reeling from Effects of Climate Change, Alaskan Village Votes to Relocate. *New York Times,* August 19.

Michener, J. (1988). *Alaska.* New York: Fawcett Crest.

Middleton-Moz, J. (1999, May 24–26). Workshop: From legacy to choice-healing the effects of generational trauma and effects on individuals, families and communities. Bloomington, MN.

Mihesuah, D. A. (1993). Suggested Guidelines for Institutions with Scholars Who Conduct Research on American Indians. *American Indian Culture and Research Journal*, 17 (3), 131–139.

Miller, J. B. (1976). *Toward a New Psychology of Women*. Boston, MA: Beacon Press.

Miller, W. R. and Rollnick, S. (2002). *Motivational Interviewing*. New York: The Guilford Press.

Mitchell, J. T. (1983). When Disaster Strikes . . . The Critical Incident Stress Debriefing Process. *Journal of Emergency Medical Services*, 8 (1), 36–39.

Mitchell, J. T. (1988). The History, Status and Future of Critical Incident Stress Debriefings. *Journal of Emergency Medical Services*, November, 47–52.

Mitchell, J.T. (2003). Major misconceptions in crisis intervention. *International Journal of Emergency Mental Health*, 5 (4), 185–197.

Mitchell, J. T. (2004). Characteristics of Successful Early Intervention Programs. *International Journal of Emergency Mental Health*, 6 (4), 175–184.

Mohatt, G., Fok, C., Henry, D. and Allen, J. (2014). Feasibility of a Community Intervention for the Prevention of Suicide and Alcohol Abuse with Yup'ik Alaska Native Youth: The Elluam Tungiinun and Yupiucimta Asvairtuumallerkass Studies. *American Journal of Community Psychology*, 54 (0), 153–169.

Mohatt, G., Hazel, K., Allen, J., Stachelrodt, M., Hensel, C. and Fath, R. (2004). Unheard Alaska: Culturally Anchored Participatory Action Research on Sobriety with Alaska Natives. *American Journal of Community Psychology*, 33 (3–4), 263–273.

Mohatt, G., Rasmus, S., Thomas, L., Allen, J., Hazel, K. and Marlatt, G. A. (2007). Risk, Resilience, and Natural Recovery: A Model of Recovery from Alcohol Abuse for Alaska Natives. *Addiction*, 103, 205–215.

Morehouse, D. (1996). *The Psychic Warrior*. New York: St. Martin's Press.

Morris, N. (2018). This Secret Experiment Tricked Psychiatrists into Diagnosing Sane People As Having Schizophrenia. *Washington Post*, January 1.

Napoleon, H. (1996). *Yuuyaraq: The Way of the Human Being*. Fairbanks, AK: University of Alaska Fairbanks.

Neihardt. J. (1932). *Black Elk Speaks*. New York: Morrow.

Nelson, S. H., McCoy, G. F., Stetter, M. and Vanderwagen, W. C. (1992). An Overview of Mental Health Services for American Indians and Alaska Natives in the 1990s. *Hospital and Community Psychiatry*, 43, (3), 257–261.

References

Norcross, J. C. (Ed.). (2001). Empirically Supported Therapy Relationships: Summary Report of the Division 29 Task Force. *Psychotherapy, 38* (4), 19–24.

Norcross, J. C. (Ed.). (2002). *Psychotherapy Relationships That Work: Therapist Contributions and Responsiveness to Patient Needs.* New York: Oxford University Press.

O'Neill, D. (1994). *The Firecracker Boys.* New York: St. Martin's Press.

Ouimette, P. C., Brown, P. J. and Najavits, L. M. (1998). Course and Treatment of Patients with Both Substance Use and Posttraumatic Stress Disorders. *Addictive Behaviors, 23* (6), 785–795.

Pack, M. J. (2012). Critical Incident Stress Debriefing: An Exploratory Study of Social Workers' Preferred Models of CISM and Experiences of CISD in New Zealand. *Social Work in Mental Health, 10,* 273–293.

Pember, M. A. (2016). Intergenerational Trauma: Understanding Natives' Inherited Pain. *Indian Country Today Media Network.*

Pewewardy, C. (2002). Learning Styles of American Indian/Alaska Native Students: A Review of the Literature and Implications for Practice. *Journal of American Indian Education, 41* (3), 22–56.

Plested, B. A., Jumper-Thurman, P. and Edwards, R. W. (2016). *Community Readiness Manual.* Fort Collins, CO: The National Center for Community Readiness, Colorado State University.

Pranis, K., Stuart, B. and Wedge, M. (2003). *Peacemaking Circles: From Conflict to Community.* St. Paul, MN: Living Justice Press.

Procyk, A. (2018). *Nutritional Treatments to Improve Mental Health Disorders.* Eau Claire, WI: PESI Publishing & Media, PESI, Inc.

Raiker, J. S., Freeman, A. J., Perez-Algorta, G., Frazier, T. W., Findling R. L. and Youngstrom, E. A. (2017). Accuracy of Achenbach Scales in the Screening of Attention-Deficit/Hyperactivity Disorder in a Community Mental Health Clinic. *Journal of the American Academy of Child and Adolescent Psychiatry, 56* (5), 401–409.

Reimer, C. S. (1999). *Counseling the Inupiat Eskimo.* Westport, CT: Greenwood Press.

Reimer, C. S. (2002). *What Is the Relationship of Suicide, Alcohol Abuse, and Spirituality Among the Inupiat?* Fairbanks, AK: University of Alaska.

Riddell, K. and Clouse, M. (2004). Comprehensive Psychosocial Emergency Management Promotes Recovery. *International Journal of Emergency Mental Health, 6* (3), 135–145.

Robjant, K. and Fazel, M. (2010). The Emerging Evidence for Narrative Exposure Therapy: A Review. *Clinical Psychology Review, 30* (8), 1030–1039.

Roesch, E. P. (1990). *Ashana.* New York: Random House.

Rogers, P. & Bloom, R. (2019). *Emotional freedom techniques and tapping for beginners*. Salisbury, England: Hope Books LTD.

Romano, J. L. (2015). *Prevention Psychology*. Washington, D.C.: American Psychological Association.

Rosenhan, D. (1973). On Being Sane in Insane Places. *Science, 179* (4070), 250–258.

Saleebey, D. (1997). *The Strengths Perspective in Social Work Practice*. Boston: Allyn and Bacon.

Saleebey, D. (2006). *The Strengths Perspective in Social Work Practice*. Boston: Pearson Education, Inc.

Scales, P. C. (2011). Youth Developmental Assets in Global Perspective: Results from International Adaptations of the Developmental Assets Profile. *Child Indicators Research, 4*, 619–645.

Scales, P. C., Benson, P. L., Dershem, L., Fraher, K., Makonnen, R., Nazneen, S., Syvertsen, A. K. and Titus, S. (2013). Building Developmental Assets to Empower Adolescent Girls in Rural Bangladesh: Evaluation of Project Kishoree Kontha. *Journal of Research on Adolescence, 23* (1), 171–184.

Schank, J. A. (1998). Ethical Issues in Rural Counselling Practice. *Canadian Journal of Counseling, 32* (4), 270–283.

Schnabel, J. (1997). *Remote Viewers*. New York: Dell Publishing.

Schon, D. A. (1987). *Educating the Reflective Practitioner*. San Francisco: John Wiley and Sons, Inc.

Schuhmann, E. M., Foote, R. C., Eyberg, S. M., Boggs, S. R. and Algina, J. (2010). Efficacy of Parent-Child Interaction Therapy: Interim Report of a Randomized Trial with Short-Term Maintenance. *Journal of Clinical Child Psychology, 27* (1), 34–45.

Search Institute. (1998). *Helping Kids Succeed—Alaskan Style*. Minneapolis, MN: Search Institute.

Sebastian, B. and Nelms, J. (2017). The Effectiveness of Emotional Freedom Techniques in the Treatment of Posttraumatic Stress Disorder: A Meta-Analysis. *Explore, (13)* (1), 16–25.

Siegel, D.J. (1999). *The developing mind*. New York: The Guilford Press.

Siegel, D. J. (2010). *The Mindful Therapist*. New York: W. W. Norton and Company.

Skewes, M. C. and Lewis, J. P. (2016). Sobriety and Alcohol Use Among Rural Alaska Native Elders. *International Journal of Circumpolar Health, 75*.

Slawinski, T. (2005). A Strengths-Based Approach to Crisis Response. *Journal of Workplace Behavioral Health, 21* (2), 79–88.

Smith, L. T. (1999). *Decolonizing Methodologies*. Dunedin, New Zealand: University of Otago Press.

Smokowski, P., Evans, C., Cotter, C. and Webber, K. (2014). Ethnic Identity and Mental Health in American Indian Youth: Examining Mediation Pathways through Self-Esteem, and Future Optimism. *Journal of Youth and Adolescence, 43* (3), 343–355.

Stahl, S. M. (2009). Epigenetics and Methylomics in Psychiatry. *Journal Of Clinical Psychiatry, 70* (9), 1204–1205.

Stahl, S. M. (2010). Fooling Mother Nature: Epigenetics and Novel Treatments for Psychiatric Disorders. *Cns Spectrum, 15* (6), 358–365.

Substance Abuse and Mental Health Services Administration. (2019). *Enhancing Motivation for Change in Substance Use Disorder Treatment*. Treatment Improvement Protocol (TIP) Series No. 35. Samhsa Publication No. Pep19-02-01-003. Rockville, MD: Substance Abuse and Mental Health Services Administration.

Sue, S. and Zane, N. (1987). The Role of Culture and Cultural Techniques in Psychotherapy: A Critique and Reformulation. *American Psychologist, 42*, 37–45.

Swisher, K. G. (1990). Cooperative Learning and the Education of American Indian/Alaska Native Students: A Review of the Literature and Suggestions for Implementation. *Journal of American Indian Education, 29* (2), 36–43.

Szyf, M., McGowan, P., Meaney, M. (2008). *The social environment and the epigenome*. Environmental and Molecular Mutagenesis, 49, 46–60.

Tamis-Lemonda, C. S., Way, N., Hughes, D., Yoshikawa, H., Kalman, K. R. and Niwa, E. Y. (2008). Parents' Goals for Children: The Dynamic Coexistence of Individualism and Collectivism in Cultures and Individuals. *Social Development, 17* (1) 183–209.

Thomason, T. (2011). Recommendations for Counseling Native Americans: Results of a Survey. *Journal of Indigenous Research, 1* (2), 1–10.

Trimble, J. E., Fleming, C. M., Beauvais, F. and Jumper-Thurman, P. (1996). Essential Cultural and Social Strategies for Counseling Native American Indians. In: Pedersen, P. B., Druguns, J. G., Lonner, W. J. and Trimble, J. E. (Eds.) *Counseling Across Cultures* (4th Ed.). Thousand Oaks, CA: Sage Publications, 177–209.

Trimble, J. E. (2010). The Virtues of Cultural Resonance, Competence, and Relational Collaboration with Native American Indian Communities: A Synthesis of the Counseling and Psychotherapy Literature. *The Counseling Psychologist, 38* (2), 243–256.

U.S. Department of Health and Human Services. (2010). *To Live to See the Great Day That Dawns: Preventing Suicide by American Indians and Alaska Native Youth and Young Adults*. DHHS Publication SMA (10)-4480, CMHS-NSPL-0196, Printed 2010. Rockville, MD: Center for Mental Health Services, Substance Abuse and Mental Health Services Administration.

Vandegraft, D. L. (1993). *Project Chariot: Nuclear Legacy of Cape Thompson*. In the *Proceedings of the U.S. Interagency Arctic Research Policy Committee Workshop on Arctic Contamination, Session A: A Native People's Concerns About Arctic Contamination II: Ecological Impacts*, May 6. Anchorage, AK: U.S. Fish and Wildlife Service.

Vazquez, C., Hervas, G., Rahona, J. and Gomez, D. (2009). Psychological Well-Being and Health. Contributions of Positive Psychology. *Annuary of Clinical and Health Psychology*, 5, 15–27.

Versluis, A. (1992). *Sacred Earth: The Spiritual Landscape of Native America*. Rochester, VT: Inner Traditions International Limited.

Waite, W. and Holder, M. (2003). Assessment of the Emotional Freedom Technique. *Scientific Review of Mental Health Practice*, 2 (1), 1–10.

Walker, C. (2014). *Behind the Dark Walls*. Instantpublisher. Com.

Waller, M. (2006). Strengths of Indigenous Peoples (Chapter 3). In Saleebey, D. (Ed.), *The Strengths Perspective in Social Work Practice*. Boston: Pearson Education, Inc.

Wall to Wall Television. (1995). *The Real X Files* (Television Documentary). London, England: Channel Four Television Company.

Wexler, L. M., Dam, H. T., Silvius, K., Mazziotti, J. and Bamikole, I. (2016). Protective Factors of Native Youth: Findings from a Self-Report Survey in Rural Alaska. *Journal of Youth Studies*, 19 (3), 358–373.

Whitfield, C. L. (2006). *Healing the Child Within*. Deerfield Beach, FL: Health Communications, Inc.

Whitfield, C. L. (2010). *Boundaries and Relationships*. Deerfield Beach, FL: Health Communications, Inc.

World Health Organization, War Trauma Foundation and World Vision International. (2011). *Psychological First Aid: Guide for Field Workers*. Geneva, Switzerland: World Health Organization.

Winkelman, M. (1994). Cultural Shock and Adaptation. *Journal of Counseling and Development*, 73 (2), 121–126.

Woititz, J. G. (1983). *Adult Children of Alcoholics*. Deerfield Beach, FL: Health Communications, Inc.

Wolf, A. S. (1989). The Barrow Studies: An Alaskan's Perspective. *American Indian and Alaska Native Mental Health Research*, 2 (3), 35–40.

Wolsko, C., Lardon, C., Hopkins, S. and Ruppert, E. (2006). Conceptions of Wellness Among the Yup'ik of the Yukon-Kuskokwim Delta: The Vitality of Social and Natural Connection. *Ethnicity and Health*, *11* (4), 345–363.

Wolynn, M. (2016). *It Didn't Start with You*. New York: Viking.

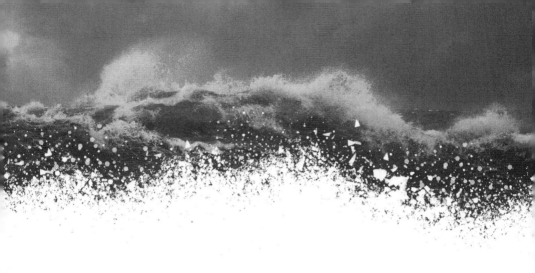

Index

Note: page numbers in italics refer to figures. Those followed by **t** refer to tables

ANTHC. *See* Alaska Native Tribal
Health Consortium
anxiety
case study, 59–64
and emotional regulation, benefits
of learning, 137–38
genetic causes of, 136
as symptom of underlying trauma,
21, 29, 45
APA. *See* American Psychological
Association
Arctic Natives, impact of global
warming on, 27–28
ASEBA. *See* Achenbach System of
Empirically Based Assessment
assertiveness, return of, with
improved mood, 62
Assets Study, 121–23, *144*
assimilation efforts, trauma of, 22
boarding schools and, 22, 31, 58
and treatment of Alaska Natives,
150
authenticity, building of, in therapy
process, 47

B

Barrow Alcohol Study, 99
Beck Depression Inventory, 60
Behavioral Health Academic Review
Committee (BHARC), 13
Behavioral Health Aide (BHA)
Program
goals of, ix
grounding in culturally sensitive
values, 13
introduction of, 12
services offered by, 12–13
behavioral health aides (BHAs)
effectiveness of
vs. mental health professionals,
14
necessity of respecting, 14–15

behavioral health aides (*continued*)
levels of certification, 12–13
as predominantly Native, ix
and prevention, 145
training programs for, 13
as village-based, ix
behavioral health practitioners
(BHPs)
as highest level of BHA
certification, 12–13
and prevention, 145
Berg, I., 77–78, 114
Bergquist, P., 22
Bering Strait region
mix of counselors and mental
health professionals working
in, x
Native communities, number and
size of, x
Nome as BHA hub for, x
Berry, J. W., 118–19
BHA program. *See* Behavioral
Health Aide (BHA) Program
BHARC. *See* Behavioral Health
Academic Review Committee
BHAs. *See* behavioral health aides
BHPs. *See* behavioral health
practitioners
bibliotheraphy, 86, *144*
Black Elk Speaks (Nieihardt), 117
boarding schools, trauma inflicted on
students in, 22, 31, 58
Boehm Test of Basic Concepts,
135–36
boundaries
healthy, importance of, 90, 112,
129
as issue in small communities, 130
See also codependence
Boundaries and Relationships
(Whitfield), 90
breathing control
as emotional regulation strategy,
49–50, 61

breathing control (*continued*)
    as frightening to some clients, 50
    and mindfulness, 43
Brockie, Teresa, 24, 137
Buber, Martin, 30
burnout in mental health
    professionals
    resistance from clients and,
      138–40
    strategies for avoiding, 141–42
B vitamins, in treatment of
    depression, 137

C

Calricaraq program, 102
Carroll, James, 22
Carved from the Heart (1997 film),
    102
case studies of psychotherapy using
    4Rs, 59–68
    depression, anxiety, and self-
      destructive ideation, 59–64
    drug and alcohol abuse, 64–68
Catholic Church, and sexual abuse of
    Native children, 21–22
CBPR. *See* community-based
    participatory research
CBT. *See* cognitive behavioral
    therapy
change
    possibility of, 150–51
    stages of (DiClemente and
      Velasquez), 139
childhood trauma, and MTHRF
    polymorphisms, 136
children
    as parent's motivation for
      recovery, 58–59, 64, 148
    separation anxiety, treatment of,
      108–9
    trauma-focused narrative therapy
      for, 80–81

Children Left Behind (Giago), 22
Christians
    and denigration of Native culture,
      20–21, 124
    and sexual abuse of Native
      children, 21–22
CISD. *See* critical incident stress
    debriefing
cities, move to, and acculturative
    stress, 120–21
codependence
    definition and characteristics of,
      111
    in health care professionals, and
      over-zealous treatment, 90,
      112
cognitive behavioral therapy (CBT),
    53, 55–56
collaboration with client
    on choice to use psychotropic
      medication, 84, 85–86
    in diagnostic labeling, 98
    on therapeutic goals, 39
    See also co-participation and
      background presence;
      self-determination of Alaska
      Natives
collaborative research methods, 100
collectivism in Alaska Native culture,
    32–33, *144*
    importance of working within, 16
    mingling with Western
      individualism, 33
    and wellness, 32
college attendance, and acculturative
    stress, 119–20
colonial language, as ongoing
    colonization, 94–95
colonization
    and damage to natural
      environment, Native
      spirituality and, 115
    definition of, 93
    existing patterns of, 93–101, *144*

Doyle, T. P., 21
Droby, Ray M.
  Alaska Native patients of, as all
    significantly stressed, 45
  and coronavirus, 23
  enjoyment of rural life in Alaska,
    18
  experience in Bering Strait
    region, x
  and mindset for treatment of
    Alaska Natives, 149–50
  nearly-fatal canoe trip in heavy
    seas, 1–7
    lessons learned in, 4–5, 7–8
  New Year's dinner with Iñupiat
    community, 73
  research by, 44–45, 53
drug abuse in Alaska Natives
  case studies, 59–64
  as cause of parent's emotionally
    unavailability, 57
  decline in, with improved mood,
    62
  and depression, 85
  and relationship with drugs rather
    than people, 148–49
  as symptom of underlying trauma,
    27, 45, 52, 61
  See also substance abuse
DSM. *See Diagnostic and Statistical
  Manual of Mental Disorders*
Duncan, B. L., 56–57, 76
Duran, B., 58–59
Duran, E., 18, 25, 58–59, 99, 107,
  147

E

Eat Right, Feel Right (Korn), 86
education, and dialogic
  communication, 30
EFT. *See* emotional freedom
  technique

ego strength, building in therapy
  process, 46–48
Elders, Native
  alcohol abuse prevention for, 101
  factors promoting successful aging
    in, 101
  importance of respect for wisdom
    of, 19–20
EMDR. *See* eye movement
  desensitization reprocessing
emotional and behavioral
  functioning, psychological tests
  for, 133
emotional freedom technique (EFT),
  50–51
  in emotional regulation, 61
  for treatment of PTSD, 54
emotional regulation
  benefits for disorders associated
    with ACEs, 137–38
  definition of, 48
  lack of, in parents, and emotional
    unavailability, 58
  learning of
    and recovery of traumatic
      memories, 58, 61, 66–67,
      112
    and reduced impact of distress,
      62, 67
  strategies for, 61, 62
  teaching of
    Action Plan in, 49–50, *51*
    case study, 66
    as goal of narrative exposure
      therapy, 54–55
    similarity to author's ocean
      canoe experience, 44,
      48–51
    stress release techniques in,
      49–51
empathy, importance to therapeutic
  relationship, 38
empowerment of Alaska Natives
  critical consciousness and, 30–32

F

G

H

mental health professionals
(*continued*)
  openness toward learning,
    17–18
  positive attitude about Native
    communities, 18, 20
  motivations, importance of self-
    awareness about, 112–13
  multifaceted role of, 15–16, *144*
  as often non-native, x
  overzealous, potential harm done
    by, 4–5
  rush to pathologize people, 96
  self-care, importance of, 141–42,
    144
  similarity of work to author's
    ocean canoe experience,
    147–48
  theoretical knowledge of, as less
    valuable than local cultural
    knowledge, 14
  and Western worldview as barrier
    to effectiveness, 107–10,
    144
  See also psychotherapy with
    Alaska Natives; treatment
    for Alaska Natives,
    guidelines for
methylenetetrahydrofolate reductase
  (MTHFR) gene, 136–37
micronutrients, in treatment of
  depression, 137
Mihesuah, D. A., 99
Miller, Jean Baker, 35
Miller, S. D., 56–57
Miller, W. R., 138–39
Millon Clinical Multiaxial Inventory,
  134
mindfulness
  breathing and, 43
  and neural integration, 41
  teaching to clients, 41
  in treatment of Alaska Natives,
    149–50

Minnesota Multiphasic Personality
  Inventory—2nd Edition
  (MMPI-2), 134
miracle question, 77
Mitchell, J. T., 82, 83
Mitnick, D. G., 50
MMPI-2. *See* Minnesota Multiphasic
  Personality Inventory—2nd
  Edition
MTHFR (methylenetetrahydrofolate
  reductase) gene, 136–37

N

Napoleon, Harold, 22, 55, 86,
  106–7
narrative exposure therapy (NET)
  available options for
    administering, 54
  benefits of, 54–55
  case study, 61–64
  conditions necessary for
    administering, 54
  precautions for use of, 55–56
  range of uses for, 54
  for trauma in Alaska Natives,
    53–54
  See also 5-Narrative CBT Model
    (Gentry); trauma-focused
    narrative therapy for
    children
National Epidemiologic Survey on
  Alcohol and related Conditions
  (Grant), 136
National Health Service Corps,
  and student loan repayment,
  18
Native Americans
  and epigenetic health disparities,
    137
  psychotherapy with, research on,
    44
  and remote viewing, 117

O

P

R

self-soothing methods. *See* emotional
regulation
separation anxiety in children,
treatment of, 108–9
Sex, Priests, and Secret Codes
(Doyle, Spie and Wall), 21
sexual abuse of Native children
books useful for addressing, 87
by Catholic priests, 21–22
and lost memories of childhood,
48, 66–67
recovered memory of, after
therapy, 66–67
sexual promiscuity, higher percentage
in subjects with ACEs, 53
Shishmaref, Alaska, relocation due to
global warming, 27
Shohet, R., 113
Shuswap people, and community
healing, 140–41, 150
Siegel, D. J., 40–41, 43
The Silence (2011 documentary),
21–22
Sipe, A. W., 21
Slawinski, T., 83
Smith, Jada, 104
Smith, Tuhiwai, 98–101
smoking, higher percentage in
subjects with ACEs, 53
social injustice
addressing through relational-
cultural therapy, 36
psychological effects of, 36
solution-focused therapy, 77
somatic problems, case study,
59–64
spirituality, Native, 115–18, *144*
colonialism's assault on, 115
and personality functioning tests,
134
and personal well-being, 115
premonitions and remote viewing,
116–17
reverence for Earth in, 115

spirituality, Native (*continued*)
spiritual visitations, 116–17
and traditional practices,
reverence for, 115–16
stages of change (DiClemente and
Velasquez), 139
sterilizations and abortions, forced,
25–26
stigma of mental health problems,
as obstacle to Native mental
health care, 128
Stiver, Irene, 35
strengths of Alaska Native
communities
generosity and strong bonds as, 73
importance of appreciating,
19–20, *144*
strengths perspective, 72–79, *144*
and critical incident stress
debriefing, 83
vs. diagnostic labeling, 97, 98
elements of, 79, 81
vs. medical/rehabilitative models,
73–76, *75t*
and motivational interviewing, 79
questions asked in, 77–79
and self determination, 74, 76,
77, 79
and solution-focused therapy, 77
techniques in, 76–79
stress release
though breathing regulation,
49–50
through emotional freedom
technique (EFT), 50–51
Stuart, B., 106
Substance Abuse and Mental Health
Services Administration
(SAMHSA)
*Enhancing Motivation for
Change in Substance Use
Disorder Treatment* (2019),
139
suicide prevention grants, 101

T

therapeutic relationship (*continued*)
　and listening skills, importance
　　of, 38
　PART acronym and, 42
　as sometimes overlooked, 46
　vital importance of, 45–46
TOVA. *See* Test of Variables of
　Attention
Toward a New Psychology of Women
　(Miller), 35
traditional knowledge and practices,
　use in treatment for Alaska
　Natives, 16
transference issues, in approach to
　Alaska Natives, 18–19, *144*
trauma-focused cognitive-behavioral
　therapy, 80–81
trauma-focused narrative therapy for
　children, 80–81, *144*
trauma in Vietnam War veterans,
　long-term effects of, 7
trauma of Alaska Natives
　ACE questionnaire in
　　identification of, 52
　behavioral effects of, 25
　epigenetic effects of, 24
　giving voice to, benefits of, 55
　high levels of, 52
　high rates of suicides and, 23
　high rates of traumatic deaths
　　and, 23–24
　manifestation in variety of
　　symptoms, 29, 40, 52
　native self-determination as only
　　solution to, 106–7
　perpetuation of, through culture
　　of silence, 28–32
　recovered memories of, after
　　learning emotional
　　regulation, 58, 66–67, 71, 112
　relational-cultural theory as best
　　approach to, 35, 36
　and resistance to treatment, 4, 7
　as treatable, 7–8

trauma of Alaska Natives (continued)
　See also ACE questionnaire;
　　colonization, Alaska Native
　　trauma from
trauma of mental health worker,
　avoiding transfer onto clients,
　149
traumatic deaths, high rates among
　Alaska Natives, 23–24
treatment for Alaska Natives
　co-participation and background
　　presence as best practice,
　　13–15, 26, *144*
　decentralized mental health
　　services as preferable,
　　12–13, *144*
　expanded thinking required in, 16
　flexibility needed in, ix, x–xi, 16
　and generalist orientation,
　　importance of, 110, *144*
　guidelines for, 9–16
　humility and, 147
　patience in, 8
　research applicable to, 37–44
　role of mental health professional
　　as multifaceted and
　　collectively mindful in,
　　15–16, *144*
　and self determination as
　　inalienable right, 10–11
　similarity to author's ocean canoe
　　experience, 147–49
　stigma of mental health problems
　　and, 128
　successful cases
　　common features of, 148
　　and resilience of human spirit,
　　149
　and traditional knowledge and
　　practices, 16
　as valuable also for Native mental
　　health providers, 9–10
　See also cultural considerations
　　in treatment for Alaska

U

V

W

Y

Z

About the Author

Ray M. Droby, Ph.D., CAPT USPHS, is a licensed psychologist who has been in the field of mental health for nearly 30 years. He has served for over 23 years in the Commissioned Corps of the U.S. Public Health Service (USPHS) in the Indian Health Service (IHS)—devoting his entire Commissioned Corps career with the tribal agency of the Norton Sound Health Corporation (NSHC). His interests in rural Alaska have included living and working in four Alaska Native communities within the Bering Strait region in addition to working and living in the multi-cultural hub community of Nome. The Norton Sound Health Corporation published his book, *With the Wind and the Waves*, in 2000—inspired by his experiences in rural Alaska. The current publication is a significant expansion of his initial work, broadened by an additional two decades of living and working in rural Alaska. Currently the director of psychological services at one of NSHC's clinics, Dr. Droby has worked with all age groups and with a variety of presenting mental health issues. His paper, *Suicide: A Human Problem*, published by *The Nome Nugget* in 2017, reflects his interest in poignant mental health problems not only within rural Alaska but nationally as well. Dr. Droby received the Cultural Humanitarian Award from the Alaska Psychological Association in 2015. In 2017, he was the recipient of the American

Psychological Association (APA) Excellence in Rural Psychology Award. He also was the 2017 recipient of the Ann Schumacher Rural Clinical Practice Award with the National Association for Rural Mental Health.